T0220303

A SIMPLE GUIDE TO

DEPRESSION

LEARNING THE BASICS

BY

W EDISON HOUPT JR MD

iUniverse, Inc.
NEW YORK   BLOOMINGTON

A Simple Guide to Depression

iUniverse books may be ordered through booksellers or by contacting:

iUniverse
1663 Liberty Drive
Bloomington, IN 47403
www.iuniverse.com
1-800-Authors (1-800-288-4677)

ISBN: 978-1-4502-2881-7 (sc)
ISBN: 978-1-4502-2882-4 (ebk)

Printed in the United States of America

iUniverse rev. date: 5/20/2010

Other books by this author:

Everyone's Everyday Guide to Practical Psychiatry

Defeating Depression

(i·Universe Publishers)

Any resemblances between the case studies and
real people are purely coincidental. These are
all fictionalized and/or amalgamated characters.

This book is not intended to diagnose or
treat any medical conditions.

Readers, who want expanded information on Depression,
will find it in my second book, *Defeating Depression*.

This book is for my family
who are curious about
the in's and out's of
direct patient care

CONTENTS

• • • • •

Please note these special terms used in this book:
(The first two words are general terms and are not capitalized whereas the next three are specific terms *only in this book* and are written with a capital "D"):

"depression" refers to the concept of sadness used in everyday speech
"depressed" means "sad"
"Depression" refers to the formal diagnosis of clinical Depression
"Depressed" describes a state of Depression in a person
"Depressive" is a Depressed person

"chronic"—a chronic psychiatric condition lasts for many years or a lifetime
"brain hormone" is a natural chemical in our brain that has anti-depressant properties (for example: serotonin, dopamine, norepinephrine, and others; the proper medical term for "brain hormone" is "neurotransmitter")
"medication" means prescription medicines (R_x medicines)

• • • • •

"Provider" refers to any mental health professional who provides service: this includes psychiatrists, psychoanalysts, psychologists, counselors, and psychotherapists (psychotherapists are also called "therapists")
Therapists, Psychologists, and **Counselors** provide service to **Clients,** whereas **Psychiatrists** provide service to **Patients**; in other words, psychiatrists have patients, and other providers have clients.
"Meg" and **"Marc"** are sometimes used "generically" throughout the book to refer to examples of gender-matched patients; this sounds less cold and clinical instead of referring to every case as "the patient" or "the client."
Otherwise, Names of specific people, such as **Sasha** actually refer to the story of that specific person (Sasha, in this case); for particulars on such a case, look up the story of that person in Part Two.

• • • • •

Other Terms, Abbreviations, and Definitions
are listed at the end of the book

• • • • •

~PREFACE~

The purpose of this book is to inform readers about the effects of Depression which is a common disorder afflicting millions of Americans. As such, this is a self-help book, not a self-diagnosis book, and it is intended for a general adult population of readers who are interested in learning the basics about Depression.

The reader of this book may be someone who has already been diagnosed with such a disorder. Such a person may wish to gain a better grasp on his feelings and situation. Another kind of reader might be wondering if he is suffering from symptoms of Depression. This kind of reader should not jump to hasty conclusions as this is not a self-diagnosis book. Notable, however, are the facts that a significant percentage of American adults do have Depression and a significant percentage of adults have had Depression symptoms at least once in their lives. Another type of reader may be a family member or friend who is concerned about someone he knows, who is battling symptoms similar to those listed in this book—or who has already been diagnosed with Depression. This type of reader may wish to obtain general background information that is of value for encouraging that someone to seek professional help or for providing emotional support for that someone's ongoing recovery. These types of readers may gain insight into the whole process of dealing with treated and untreated Depression. And, some readers may merely be interested in learning more about Depression for whatever reason.

SPECIFICS ABOUT THE AUTHOR

I did my training at the Cleveland Clinic and continued to work in Cleveland, Ohio, for almost another decade. I worked in the hospital, outpatient clinics, and in the regional Psychiatric Emergency

Room at St. Vincent Charity Hospital in downtown Cleveland. I am interested in Mood Disorders, Emergency Psychiatry, Sleep Disorders, and psychiatric disorders of medical patients (Consultation-Liaison Psychiatry).

I have been working in Southern California for the last decade doing Consultation-Liaison Psychiatry and office psychiatry in Los Angeles, as well as geriatric psychiatry in numerous local nursing homes in the eastern half of Los Angeles County. In San Bernardino County, I worked in the County's clinic system (specifically, in Nueva Vida Clinic in Colton, CA).

SPECIFICS ABOUT THIS BOOK

This book is divided into three Parts. Part One presents basic background information about Depression. Part Two presents the fictionalized but realistic stories ("case histories") about people who become Depressed. The cases may show how, when, and why people might become Depressed. As far as who becomes Depressed, this can happen to almost anyone. The stories range from simple cases to moderately complicated cases (the reader who wants to read about quite complicated cases can read these in my book *Defeating Depression*). This book describes the basic process of diagnosing patients and treating disorders.

The treatment of real patients is based on textbook information and clinical experience. The practical aspects of diagnosis and treatment are called clinical experience (art of medicine), whereas textbook information is based on medical knowledge, scientific research, and updates in the medical sciences. There is no bibliography of references for the core information in this book. The reader may thus consider this book to belong to a special genre of "creative non-fiction." Perhaps, an alternate description of the genre of this book could be that of "observational psychiatry," in other words, based on my observations of human behavior over the past thirty years. When references were consulted, most of the information was extracted (and cited) from standard authorities such as: Kaplan and Sadock's *Comprehensive Textbook of Psychiatry* (2,084 pages), the *DSM-IV-TR*, the *PDR (Physicians Desk Reference)*, Steven Stahl's *Essentials of Psychopharmacology, Basic and Clinical Pharmacology* by Bertram Katzung, *Goodman and Gilman's Pharmacological Basis of Therapeutics,* Jerrold Bernstein's *Drug Therapy in Psychiatry,* and others. There is no bibliography at the end of this book.

Edison Houpt
Pasadena, California
July, 2010

PART ONE

DEFINING AND DESCRIBING DEPRESSION

BACK-STORY OF DEPRESSION
WHAT IS DEPRESSION?
WHAT ARE ITS CAUSES AND
ORIGINS?

BACK-STORY

How nice it would be to write about the kinds of Depression, but unfortunately, Depression is not kind, so I write instead about the types of Depression. Depression is unkind in that it does not respect age, gender, social class, financial status, or any other boundaries. Depression is unkind because it affects many aspects of a person's life, and not just mood; it also affects activity levels, sleep, hunger, concentration, attention span, motivation, enjoyment, sexual desire, and interpersonal relations. Then, after negatively affecting some or all of these aspects of life, Depression moves on to highjack basic survival skills and instincts.

Depression is not seductive like alcoholism and compulsive disorders, but rather overtakes its victims by suppressing their abilities to recognize its slow onset—in most cases—and thereby takes control of its victims slyly and gradually. Day after day, Marc or Meg may feel slightly less enthusiastic about life in general. When their brains become Depressed, they slowly lose the ability to process information coming in from the outside world. And when the information does come in, the Depressed brain processes the information more slowly. Slowly, less and less information trickles in, and when it does, it is processed more slowly. A tired and Depressed brain is a slowed brain, so the Depressed brain is slow in sending out responses, also. There is a general overall

3

slowing, but Marc and Meg may not notice, since everything inside and outside their minds' world view is also equally slowed. It is like a slowed person driving a car slowly—the world seems to be at speed, from his perspective. After the symptoms accumulate gradually over time, the victims will awaken one day and realize that they feel out of kilter. They conclude that something is wrong: they may come to the conclusion that they have become Depressed. Perhaps the victims can identify the feelings as Depression, but oftentimes, they cannot. The feelings may be those of lack of desire, lack of desire to do anything and lack of desire to continue striving to be someone. Marc and Meg will finally and definitively note that something is wrong, but may be unsure what is happening. Depression overtakes a person's abilities to cope with daily activities and to function normally. Depression suppresses a person's will power and puts his life on "auto-pilot," going to no place good. Home life, jobs, families, enjoyment, employment stability, pastimes, and—eventually—even personality are all assaulted by this "identity thief" called Depression.

There are other cases in which the victim is aware of the onslaught of the Depression—perhaps because she is attuned to her feelings or perhaps because the onset of the Depression is rather rapid. But in many cases, the onset is insidious, and once begun, can become relentless until treatment is sought.

Depression, as its name implies, depresses mood but even worse, it depresses its victim's ability to recognize the gravity of his gradual deterioration. Depression reduces, depresses, and slows a person's functional level. His mental and bodily activities are all slowed. A slowed mind is now in charge of analyzing the external world as well as his internal thoughts and sensations, and a mind slowed from Depression begins to function in "brown-out" mode. His tired brain is unable to process all the incoming data and mount a coordinated and reasonable response. Many of the data are disregarded and discarded because his "browned-out" brain is unable to retrieve memories needed for a meaningful response. A different situation occurs with internal sensations in which the internal nervous relay system seems to operate at reduced levels. A weakened nervous system delivers fewer incoming signals to his "browned-out" brain. He feels less "connected" to his internal feeling state. He makes fewer decisions and formulates fewer internal responses; less information is sent back to his body via the signal-weary nervous system. As the victim becomes more Depressed, he becomes more slowed and his ability to fend off the Depression weakens further. At some moments, he may have a vague realization that all is not well, and he may have breakthrough episodes of irritability, but the episodes are unfocused. Since the Depressed victim does not know how to fight this new invisible and gradually worsening foe, his irritability may give way to frustration as the Depression settles in and becomes entrenched like an emotional parasite.

Depression is classified as a Mood Disorder, but it could just as easily be called a general dysfunction disorder, or an appetite disorder. As a general dysfunction disorder, it affects most areas of life by lowering them from a normal level to a poorly functioning level. Likewise, Depression could be called an appetite disorder based on psychiatrists' understanding that food, sex, and activities are all "appetites" in the strict sense of this Latin word. Despite its suggestive name that it is a Mood Disorder, Depression is also much more. It is much more than just mere sadness. That is why I am using the term "depressed" (with a lower case "d") to mean "sad," while I am using the term "Depressed" (capital "D") to refer to the whole combination of emotional disabilities that are present in a clinical Depression. Clinical Depression is much more than sadness.

So, What is Depression?

Most people think of Depression as the popular concept of "depression," which they would define as sadness, tearfulness, or loneliness. This might be an accurate description of some mild Depressions, but this falls far short of describing many cases of Depression.

In practice, the definition of Depression could be better stated as any alteration in Meg's normal baseline behavior resulting in non-beneficial changes in her internal feeling state and in her ability to cope with the rest of the world. The result of this means that her functional level and efficiency decrease, resulting in a deterioration that is usually obvious to other people (but not always) and usually somewhat obvious to her (but not always). If the Depression continues untreated, however, the Depressive symptoms will become quite obvious to everybody—and eventually even to her. One of the key points of practical diagnosis is that her current behavior should represent a significant change (deterioration) from her previous baseline behavior. I feel that this is the cornerstone of diagnosis because it allows for comparing her past normal baseline behavior to the new onset of unproductive behavior patterns which would be considered abnormal for her—thus, Depressive.

THE BRAIN IN DEPRESSION

Our brain has structure (anatomy) and function (electro-chemical activity). The human brain is structurally three brains under one skull. We have a small primitive brain deep inside our head. This is the brain that we share with reptiles. I know, this sounds slimy—but it's true. The small primitive brain helps us with all the basic activities of life: finding food and mates, swimming, breathing, walking, and sleeping, and so on. The second brain is much better: this is the mammal brain that we share with all higher animals like dogs, pigs, and monkeys. It makes us mammals like them. The third and highest brain is our most recent brain and is the brain that makes us human. It is that which makes us more exceptional than dogs, pigs, and monkeys. This is the brain that allows us to make elaborate future plans, design machinery, graduate from high school, launch satellites, create pharmaceuticals, and so on.

As far as function of the brain, part of its activity is chemical and part is electro-chemical. The chemical part consists of important "hormones," especially "brain hormones" that keep us happy, attentive, and free of Depression and anxiety. The "brain hormones" stimulate activity in the nerve cells of the brain to produce pleasant sensations such as joy, attention, satisfaction, and well-being. The electrochemical activity is the way that the whole brain functions, which we still do not understand.

Researchers believe that low levels of the "feel-good" "brain hormones" may be linked to Depression. This is hard to study in living humans. However, these low "hormone" levels have been studied in rats. Researchers have discovered methods to raise and lower the brain hormones of rats as well as to block the effects. Unfortunately, we do not know if altered hormonal levels make rats feel Depressed or if rats are even capable of suffering from clinical Depression. The best that researchers can do is to give experimental antidepressants to hormone-depleted rats to see if the rodents become livelier. If so, then perhaps the experimental antidepressant might be effective for humans. Some of these effects in rats can be verified by observing brain hormones and antidepressants tagged with special atoms that can be seen under a microscope.

The notion that human Depression is caused by low levels of "brain hormones" is still a theory and not a proven scientific fact. Research during the twentieth century pointed to possible involvement of three main "brain hormones": dopamine, serotonin, and norepinephrine which are probably the most important ones—but we are not even completely sure of that. Researchers believe that "brain hormones" are in normal "balance" in non-Depressed people, but that the "hormones" are too low or out of balance in Depression. The popular press refers to this as "chemical imbalance." Originally, we thought that low hormone levels caused Depression, but there are other possible explanations for altered brain hormones in Depression. As of the year 2010, we know that there is a long list of brain hormones and chemicals that could be out of balance—not just these three. The only proof of this imbalance in humans is a few studies of autopsies on suicides and results from electronic PETScans of the brain. We cannot submit human brains to the same experiments used on rats.

The true nature of this chemical "imbalance" is open to speculation. We have no way to measure the "normal" levels of these "brain hormones" in humans. We have no way to prove that these altered chemical levels are the cause of anything. They may just as likely be the fall-out from the Depression which itself is caused by some other brain problem further "up-stream." In other words, some unknown factor may cause biochemical changes that result in the observed "chemical imbalance." Changes in serotonin, dopamine, and norepinephrine may be incidental markers of the Depression but not the cause of or the cure for Depression.

CAUSES

The cause of Depression in some cases may be known, but in many cases, the cause is unknown. The unknown causes occur in persons who seemingly have no reason to be Depressed; they have no Depression in the family and no risk factors. In these people, Depression seems to come from nowhere. The overall frequency of getting Depressed in this way increases with age: the older a person grows, the likelier she is to get Depressed from unknown causes. Depression of unknown cause can occur at any age; however, it noticeably starts affecting adults in their mid 30's, and then the risk increases as we age. It becomes quite common in the elderly. It can also occur before or with the onset of dementias, like Alzheimer's Dementia.

There are some cases of Depression that have known causes, and these can be divided into: biological, medical, chemical, genetic, physical, and emotional. The overall frequency of getting Depressed from known causes tends to increase with age also, as does Depression from unknown cause. However, aging is a less important risk factor in known causes; the more important risk factor comes from the causative factor itself. Certain causes are likelier to cause Depression, and among those, the more severe causes are likelier to cause a deeper Depression. For example, epilepsy and multiple sclerosis are both brain diseases. As a result, patients with either of these disorders are likelier to have Depression than a healthy person. Patients with multiple sclerosis are likelier to have episodes of Depression than epileptics. Thus, younger persons with multiple sclerosis might be at higher risk than older patients with epilepsy. The risk from known causes does not necessarily increase with age, but increases with worsening degrees of the primary cause.

Biological causes include electrocution, suffocation, or surviving a near-death experience. *Medical causes* include: neurological diseases, low hormone levels (thyroid, adrenal, pituitary, and steroid hormones), and so on. *Chemical causes* include poisons, diet pills, street drugs (Ecstasy, MDMA, crystal "meth"), daily abuse of anabolic steroids for bodybuilding, and certain prescription medications. Some common prescription medications that can cause Depression are stomach pills (Reglan, Tagamet), heart pills (Inderal), prescription steroids (Prednisone), and a number of other drugs. *Genetic causes* occur in people who have Depressed relatives as well as depressed alcoholic relatives. Some of these depressed or Depressed alcoholic relatives may even have been very Depressed and committed suicide. *Physical causes* result from structural brain damage, such as: massive brain surgery, head injuries (auto accidents and sports, especially football and boxing), and so on ("he was never quite the same again after falling off the roof"). *Emotional causes* can be the electro-chemical equivalent of physical head trauma and may result in severe emotional disturbances; these are "traumatic" Depressions, essentially a mental—but non-physical—brain injury. The ways in which emotionally traumatic events cause Depression are not specifically known, but we do know that children and teenagers who have experienced great emotional trauma are at higher risk for Depression. The physical and emotional Depressions can occur shortly after the causative event (war, car accident) or sometime later in life (boxing, sexual abuse), whereas the medical, biological, and chemical causes usually occur at the same time as the causative factor. Genetic causes may appear at any time in life, but tend to follow two general trends: if Jerrold is coming down with the same Depression that his uncles have, then he should get the Depression at about the same age that his uncles got sick. In other words, these cases of genetic Depression, are probably unleashed by a timing gene: we have timing genes in our body that turn on and off as we reach certain ages—if not, then we would never have puberty, get married, or age. A second trend in genetic Depression shows that some people will get Depressed when a certain condition occurs in their lifetime—whenever that event, occurs, then the Depression will begin. Considering all the ways to become Depressed, it is possible that in the future, more and more unknown causes may be found to have known causes.

RISK FACTORS

There are also risk factors for Depression. These risk factors do not cause Depression, but may leave a person vulnerable and more susceptible to developing a Depression that is due to known or unknown causes; such risk factors are job stress (harassment or frequent job moves), financial distress (bankruptcy), divorce, serious family problems, multiple funerals, and prolonged residence in a foreign country (especially one that is recognized as a "hardship post"). The stress associated with these risk factors can come in the form of physical stress or of non-physical stress. Physical stress would affect the body: the heart beats faster, muscles are straining, water and sodium are lost through perspiration, and so on. Physical stress may increase calcium deposits in bone, increase our core body temperature, use up stored sugar, produce red blood cells, result in sodium and water loss, and increase muscle mass. What many people may not realize is that non-physical stress can also cause biochemical changes inside the body. Examples of these non-physical stressors are: emotional, mental, spiritual, or social stress (with the understanding that economic and political stress fall within social stress). Emotional stress is demonstrated by mood reactions; mental stress is demonstrated by altered thoughts; and, spiritual stress is indicated by uneven ethics and moral codes. All these types of stress can cause biochemical stress inside our bodies—whether the stress is physical or non-physical.

However, non-physical stress may also result in other biochemical reactions inside our bodies. The results might be: altered levels of cortisol (the "stress hormone"), depleted brain hormones, and surging adrenaline causing high blood pressure. This has a further reaction that may cause us to engage in "nervous nibbling," eating too much sugar, salt, and fat that ends up stored in our body. This non-physical stress is unlike physical stress where we are consuming and losing sugar, salt, fat, and water, and possibly losing calcium or having it deposited outside the bones. Whether we are experiencing physical or non-physical stress, our body is biochemically reacting to our environment, because both physical and non-physical stresses usually come from our environment. Thus, environment can shape what we are and how we react to those environmental stress factors. (Also, see the following Section on Risk Factors.)

KNOWN CAUSES OF DEPRESSION

There are many diseases and medications that can cause Depression. Among the diseases, there are medical, neurological, and a few psychiatric disorders. Among the medications, there are dozens that are in common daily use in general medicine, neurology, and psychiatry. Here is a short list:

MEDICATIONS THAT CAN CAUSE DEPRESSION

Antipsychotic medications may cause Depression in certain people, but this is usually not a serious problem. This occurs with old medications such as Thorazine.

Chantix helps people to quit smoking, but Chantix has been reported to make people depressed, perhaps because it suppresses the "feel-good" "brain hormone," dopamine. However, quitting cigarettes results in quitting nicotine, too. Since cigarettes are highly addicting (like cocaine), some people who quit smoking, may go into mourning for the loss of the beloved addictive object: mourning equals depression. Nicotine can have mild antidepressant properties, so nicotine withdrawal by itself could cause depression. Also, some cigarette smokers are self-treating a mild Depression with cigarettes. When these people quit nicotine, the original Depression may show itself again. Thus there are varied sources of depression and Depression that could exist independently of any Chantix side effects.

Cimetidine—see Tagamet

Inderal is an older blood pressure pill. It crosses freely into the brain and can cause Depression and nightmares. In the last thirty-some years, many new blood pressure drugs have been invented that do not have this effect.

Interferon is a treatment for hepatitis. Interferon is notorious for causing Depression in normal people, let alone in Depressed people whose Depressions can worsen while on Interferon. Interferon treatment lasts for a year or more. Hepatitis patients with long-standing Depression often require antidepressants while taking hepatitis treatment. Hepatitis patients without a personal history of Depression may also need to be monitored for any first-onset Depression arising from the hepatitis treatment.

Epilepsy drugs in high doses can cause depression and Depression in some epileptics: Topamax, Dilantin, and Phenobarbital, for example.

Metoclopramide—see Reglan

Prednisone is a steroid hormone that can cause mood changes.

Propranolol—see Inderal

Prostate cancer treatments: some prostate cancer grows when exposed to male hormone. Therefore, some prostate cancer treatments focus on lowering male hormones. Low male hormones can make men feel depressed or Depressed.

Reglan—is a medication for diabetic stomach problems. If it accumulates and reaches a high blood level, it can cause Depression notable for slowing both the mind and the body.

Retinoic Acid is a dermatology preparation associated with Depressive symptoms.

Tagamet is a stomach pill that can cause Depression, especially in older men in whom it prevents the production of male hormone. Low male hormone levels can make men feel depressed.

MEDICAL DISORDERS THAT CAN CAUSE DEPRESSION

Common examples are cancer, kidney failure, chronic pain, and hormonal imbalances. Cancer patients can have varying types of Depression, most of which is due to end-of-life issues and less so, from a direct biochemical effect of the cancer. The same applies to kidney failure. Chronic pain from any cause usually results in chronic Depression; this complicated relationship is discussed in *Everyone's Everyday Guide to Practical Psychiatry, Chapter VI-5.*

Glandular organs produce hormones. Hormones are internal bio-chemicals that are made in one organ and then travel around the body to cause effects in other organs. If the glandular organs are diseased, then they may make too much or too little hormonal product. This results in hormonal imbalances that can then cause Depression. Cortisol is the "stress hormone" that is made in the adrenal glands (on top of the kidney); if cortisol levels are too high or too low, then Depression can result. There is excess cortisol in Cushing's Disease, and too little cortisol in Addison's Disease. Disease of the thyroid gland (located in the front of the neck) can cause changes in thyroid hormones, which in turn can cause behavioral changes. Low thyroid can present with weight gain, tiredness, depression or Depression, and lack of motivation. This can be offset by taking thyroid pills. Likewise, changes in the levels of pituitary gland hormones (in the brain) may result in Depression. Also, any factor that lowers male hormone levels will make men Depressed. Changes in female hormones later in life are well known to be associated with mood symptoms in women. Whenever a doctor sees a new patient with Depression, the first order of diagnosis is to verify that the patient does not have any of these medical disorders which can cause Depressive symptoms. If these new patients have Depression due to a medical disorder, then they have a Secondary Depression (the medical disorder is the primary problem). Some primary medical causes of Secondary Depression cannot be corrected (cancer, kidney failure, multiple sclerosis), so the psychiatrist must "treat around" the primary disease. Most of the glandular sources of Secondary Depression due to too high or too low hormone levels can be corrected medically by restoring hormonal balance; however, some of the medications and treatments for the primary medical problem have their own significant side effects.

NEUROLOGICAL DISORDERS CAN CAUSE DEPRESSION

In theory, any brain disorder (neurological) could cause (psychiatric) symptoms. In reality, certain brain disorders are likelier to cause Depression than others. Depression is very common in Parkinson's Disease and in Dementias (Alzheimer's). Brain tumors and brain cancer can cause dementia, confusion, psychosis, or Depression. John Travolta played the role of a man who developed extraordinary mental abilities due to brain cancer (movie *Phenomenon*). Strokes can cause Depression also. Epilepsy (Seizure disorder) can cause psychiatric symptoms— as can certain epilepsy drugs used to treat epilepsy. Many other rare neurological conditions may occur with Depression (Huntington's chorea, for example). Chronic Brain Infections—such as herpes and HIV/AIDS—can cause Depression.

Parkinson's Disease and Dementia are both brain diseases in which parts of the brain are deteriorating. This is the primary disease: this is real brain damage which can cause a secondary Depression. Also, the patients are aware that they have very serious destructive fatal brain diseases, and this knowledge alone could make anyone Depressed (called Reactive Depression). Thus, there may be three sources of Depression: one physical cause (due to structural damage of the brain), one electro-chemical cause (due to lowered levels of "brain hormones"), and the emotional reaction to the knowledge of having the disease. The physical cause is diagnosed as Parkinson's disorder or as Alzheimer's disease. The electro-chemical cause is Secondary Depression (Depression secondary to Parkinson's or Alzheimer's), and the emotional reaction is Reactive Depression.

AIDS has even more possible causes of Depression. AIDS often occurs with both dementia and Depression. The dementia provides the three already mentioned possible sources of Depression. Apart from these three, AIDS patients can also become Depressed from several other causes:

- Depression that existed before the patient turned HIV positive;
- Depression related to adjusting to a new life situation with serious revision of life plans: changing from long-term to short-term goals;

13

- Social Stigma and Ostracism: Becoming a modern leper is not likely to be an esteem-bolstering event. Social and occupational stigmatization still happens nowadays, sometimes in a less obvious way than in the movie *Philadelphia* (1993);
- Romantic disappointments: It is difficult to forge a new relationship armed with the knowledge that this is in effect a fatal venereal disease. Anyone who contemplates a relationship with an HIV positive person is at risk of contracting a fatal disease;
- Generalized fatigue with loss of interest in life;
- Depression related to medication side-effects;
- Distress about the costs of medicines (a few thousand dollars per month); and,
- Grief related to deaths and funerals of friends.

Some of these above-listed Depressions may be classified as Major Depression, Dysthymia, Reactive Depression, Minor Depression, or Secondary Depression.

OTHER PSYCHIATRIC DISORDERS THAT CAN CAUSE A SECONDARY DEPRESSION

Long-standing anxiety disorders can cause Depression by using up the "brain hormones." Three examples of such anxiety disorders are Generalized anxiety, Panic Attacks, and PTSD (Post-Traumatic Stress Disorder). Another example is the Depression that may occur with schizophrenia. This is a Secondary Depression that can occur after a major schizophrenic episode ("nervous breakdown"), called "post-psychotic Depression." A third example is found in patients with Borderline Personality Disorder who are well known for suffering from alternating waves of various types of Depression: dysphoria, Reactive Depression, and Major Depression.

BURDEN OF DEPRESSION

Major Depression is a common diagnosis seen by general psychiatrists all over the country. It occurs frequently in developed nations which spend billions of dollars each year to treat it. Depression is one of the world's leading causes for disability, sick days, and even death; death can come actively by suicide or passively by slowly wasting away. A large number of Depressed people are not working. In the wealthy nations, the patient is usually able to receive some financial support during his time off work; in other countries where idleness means hunger, the financial consequences of Depression can be harsher. Some people have lingering, smoldering, untreated mild Depressions that result in backaches, headaches, irritable bowel symptoms, asthmatic anxiety, etc. These people are able to take off a couple sick days here and there. Other Depressed workers who do not have these bodily symptoms, will have purely emotional symptoms such as those from irritable Depression or slowed Depression. Their feelings interfere with their ability to work productively. Men tend to self-treat irritable Depression with alcohol. The combination of alcohol and untreated Depression in men results in lowering their inhibitions, which means that men's anger can be provoked by trivial events and minor nuisances. And, then men start overreacting to major stress factors. Thus, men become likely to act out their emotions instead of discussing their emotions. This can cause angry outbursts and decreased sex-drive, which then makes men even angrier, so that they drink even more, and so on. Depressed women will become quite moody—or moodier and may overeat or over-shop. Overeating causes a host of new medical problems such as obesity, and over-shopping may result in marital strife (angry husbands, who hopefully, are not already Depressed themselves).

Depression can result in death directly or indirectly. The most obvious direct cause is suicide. There are also a number of indirect causes: accidents due to inattentiveness, alcoholism, forgetting to renew health insurance, loss of job and hence loss of medical insurance, starving on the streets (in poor nations), etc. Some Depressed people will deliberately refuse to seek treatment for Depression, thus resulting in a kind of passive suicidal behavior by refusing to do something that might extend the quality and duration of life. Thus, they slowly waste away: they lose weight; they are inactive so that their muscles become weak, and all the normal biochemical processes in their bodies slow down or halt. All of which also decreases resistance to infections. Furthermore, as a result of abnormal biochemical processes, normal body rhythms are disrupted. The normal rhythm of cortisol levels is disrupted (cortisol, the "stress hormone"). After this goes on for a while, Depressed people go on to develop poor sleep cycles, resulting in napping in the daytime, pacing around in the wee hours, and insomnia. People with insomnia become confused—and sometimes agitated, too—in the daytime. This is the aftermath of a slowed Depression that results in poor nutrition.

Also related possibly to abnormalities of cortisol, a slowed-down Depression can lower emotional strength and lead to the inability to face up to stress. This also makes Depressives more susceptible to the negative effects of stress, with the result that they develop physical symptoms (see "somatizing" in the Vocabulary). If these physical symptoms last for a long time, then stress-induced physical diseases occur, among which heart attack is the worst, but many others also occur, such as ulcers, headaches, and insomnia. These major medical illnesses represent the physical aspect of the Depression, resulting ultimately in death that differs little from controlled starvation. The impact of Depression on the labor pool of able-bodied adults amounts to countless billions of lost revenue dollars worldwide.

EARLY WARNING SIGNS
AND
ONSET OF DEPRESSION

Onset of Depression may be gradual, sudden, or delayed. Gradual onset accounts for most cases of Depression and these cases are usually of unknown cause. Gradual onset can take months to develop fully; sudden onset may appear within a matter of days or a week. Of course, there are some intermediate cases that may take a couple weeks or a few short weeks to develop. Typically, Depression due to hormonal imbalances or certain medications can be in the range of intermediate to gradual. Some Depression may be so gradual that it requires years to occur; these cases appear as a delayed onset Depression: Depression due to head trauma from boxing is one such example. In other cases, a Depression with very slow onset may represent the development of a Chronic Depression, which evolves slowly in a leisurely manner, and persists indefinitely.

Cases of sudden-onset Depression may be linked to one major known cause (as described above) or to a series of rather minor events which all occur within a short time period. These minor events that would not be a cause of Depression in and of themselves, may all add up to the point of equaling one known cause of Depression. This is called "kindling" effect (see Betty's story). This outcome could vary from person to person: one person might be affected by a certain collection of minor events that would not affect another. Sudden-onset Depression is less common than Depression of unknown cause.

Depression with a slow and gradual onset usually has no known cause. A person like Marc may feel a twinge that something ominous is approaching, perhaps a disturbance in his body's internal "rhythms"—

provided that he has awareness of such goings-on. The earliest onset symptoms at this point may sometimes be avoided or delayed if Marc embraces new fulfilling experiences. How can he sense the omen of this shadowy psychological possibility? Only if he has a strong inner sense, and only if he is willing to heed its early warning. Most people cannot because the slow gradual onset may be very subtle—the symptoms may appear so slowly that a person adjusts to them over time without realizing that he is slowly being dragged down. Most people are extremely distracted by all the frustrations and rush of life in our modern stressful society. People caught up on this treadmill have already sealed their fate because they are not in close contact with their inner spiritual being. They are at high risk.

The onset of Depression may be marked by Marc's inner feelings as well as outward behaviors that are observed by other people. A Depressive like Marc is usually aware of his inner feelings, but may not realize how serious they are—or what impact they have on other people. Marc may or may not be aware of how he is behaving or how other people are observing his outward behaviors. He may be partially or completely unaware of how he is upsetting or annoying other people. Part of the reason is that his brain is "browning out" so that feedback from the outside world is slowed down also. His ability to see himself as he really is, has become even more diminished than under his non-Depressed state (Marc's "observing ego" is faltering).

The feelings which he feels inside himself are symptoms. The external behaviors observed by others are called the "signs of disease," or more simply, "signs." Some of the warning symptoms and signs of an early Depression are listed here. The symptoms are listed first, and the signs are listed second (in parentheses):

- Slow decline in interest in hobbies, activities, and pastimes (avoidance)
- Noticeable decline in the quality of work at home and on the job (complaints from supervisors, teachers, and family members)
- Loss of appetite (weight loss)
- New onset of need to take naps on the weekends (spending many hours in bed isolated from friends and family)

- Cutting down on social activities (shunning visitors by staying in bedroom, decrease in the number of hours spent with people, and decrease in the amount of time spent on such activities)
- Frustration with life (irritability, outbursting, or tearfulness for no apparent reason)
- Self-medicating (drinking alcohol and buying herbal antidepressants)
- Sleep problems (pacing at night, going to bed very early, awakening in the wee hours)
- Pessimism (unwise decisions based on personalized doom-and-gloom forecasts)

As Depression continues, it will start to bat its victim around. A person like Meg may be clueless—she knows that she feels a bit "off." Likely, she cannot identify the source of the sensation, if it is her first Depression. She will think it is a menstrual problem, a virus, a medical disease, a "bad hair day," a family problem, boyfriend problem, or something else. Marc thinks perhaps if he could "bulk up" he would attract friends and thus feel better about himself; he might worry about his acne, he might plan to buy a used motorcycle or Camaro, or he might suffer due to the absence of his friend Raj who has gone off to college. Meg and Marc may spend every weekend in bed feeling unmotivated which supports a self-diagnosis of having "some virus." If Meg does not recognize an emotional Depression and thinks that it is a real medical problem, then that is called "somatizing" (see Vocabulary): these patients think that their symptoms are in their bodies and not in their heads. Family doctors think that the symptoms are in the patients' heads and not in their bodies. The truth is that all symptoms are processed in the brain, so in a sense, symptoms are always in our heads. Family doctors see a lot of mildly Depressed people who feel physically uncomfortable—these patients are Depressed, but they do not realize it. Examples of the symptoms of physical discomfort are: vague miserable and lousy feelings (lack of regular exercise), mild backache (too much time lying in bed or sitting in tension at the workplace), stomach acidity (worrying), headaches (stress), asthma attacks, and high diabetic sugar levels—to name only a few. Family doctors end up treating a lot of mildly Depressed patients, who often never see a psychiatrist.

Patients like Altagracia or Sasha who have these physical symptoms are offended if their family doctor suggests that they have a "nervous" condition, and they may not take the antidepressants that are offered. Or, the patients may take the pills for a couple days, develop the usual first-week side effects, and then refuse to try any more antidepressants. So, their minor Depressions grow worse and become Anxious Depression or Major Depression. Meanwhile, Altagracia keeps on coming back to see the family doctor with the somatizing symptoms, and she is getting worse and feeling frustrated (with the lack of definite diagnosis). Meanwhile, she is not taking prescribed antidepressants, so the family doctor is getting frustrated with her and her lack of cooperation. The next step occurs when the family doctor tells her that she must see a psychiatrist. Then she is indignant for being told that she is "mental" and blames the family doctor for diagnostic incompetence. So, patients who have their first Depression are confused, to say the least, and may not be willing to get necessary treatment.

When first-time patients like Phyllis or Florence feel sick enough to seek out professional help, they are usually in an emotionally compromised state already and have decreased decision-making capacity. A person like Enrique may feel that he has reached such a low bottom in his life, that life has little meaning or importance. Friends or family may urge him to seek treatment. Sometimes, employers insist upon it. This is the time when patients may try self-treatment. They may try herbs or turn to drugs, alcohol, or other thrills such as over-spending and over-shopping. These are all compulsive behaviors that may release feel-good brain hormones. However, these attempts at self-treatment serve only to put off the day of reckoning. As people continue to self-treat in this way, the Depression has time to fester and grow worse and worse until it becomes harder to treat. It is amazing how many people self-treat for so many months or years.

The situation should be easier if the patient is having her second Depression, but she may still be taken off guard for a few weeks, during which time her family will be just as likely to note the return of the Depression as is she. Her family may make the diagnosis first: that she is getting Depressed again.

Compulsive behaviors can also surface and get out of control. Overeating and over-shopping can become problem behaviors. Over-shopping and over-spending can result in small surges of "brain hormones" that are responses to the thrill of the pursuit and the risk of debt and all the stress involved in indebtedness (angry husbands). Overeating of sugars, salt, fats, and chemicals has definite biochemical effects on the body also. Sugar results in adrenaline surges (stimulation). Salt raises the blood pressure. Fats result in biochemical changes, and all the chemical preservatives have unknown long-term effects (abnormal calcifications?).

SYMPTOMS OF DEPRESSION

This part of the book is not intended as a form of self-diagnosis, but as a crude method of identifying any Depression that might be present. Obviously, diagnosis should be done by a licensed mental health professional. Like stress, Depression can have four categories of symptoms, which are physical, mental, emotional, and spiritual. The physical symptoms are symptoms in our bodies, "somatizing" (see Vocabulary). Emotional symptoms are demonstrated by mood reactions. Mental symptoms express themselves in altered thoughts. And, spiritual symptoms present as uneven ethics and casual moral codes. When we discuss the symptoms of Depression, we do not usually divide them up, but rather list them as shown below. Please note that psychiatrists recognize different types of appetites: food appetite, sexual appetite (called libido), sleep, and physical activity (hobbies/outside interests/pastimes). The following is a list of some of the typical symptoms (and signs) of Depression.

FOOD APPETITE

A mild loss of appetite for food is a symptom of a typical Depression. If that symptom is left untreated, it can progress into moderate weight loss. If enough weight is lost, then a state of mild starvation occurs in which the patient will become thin and malnourished—this much weight loss is not common but can occur with Severe and Psychotic Depressions. Having a slender body may not be so awful, but the worst thing for a Depressed brain is to be deprived of a diet containing energy (carbohydrates), minerals, and vitamins (especially B-complex vitamins). However, acquiring a slender body by this technique is a poor tactic that can result in muscle wasting and other problems.

Apart from losing weight, there are also Depressions in which people overeat, gain weight, and become sluggish—these have classically been considered not typical of Depression, but they are becoming commoner, possibly because of the high prevalence of overeating and obesity in America. It is becoming commoner for me to see overweight people who complain that they have lost their food appetite. This is not a serious physical condition because these people are already overweight, but they see it as a distressing symptom because it represents a great loss of pleasure (loss of food appetite and the enjoyment from overeating). In effect, this appetite loss they would classify as a lack of interest in usual fun activities. No matter how illogical these statements seem, in the sense that these same people need to lose twenty to forty pounds, this is often their main complaint about the Depression and the most distressing symptom to them. And they want this symptom corrected. This also supports my statement that Depression symptoms represent any change that a person would consider to be a change from her normal baseline behavior (enjoying food).

Decreased activity levels in typical underweight Depression is from physical wasting, whereas decreased activity in non-typical overweight Depression may be from sluggishness (see *Isolation* below).

SLEEP

Sleep is often the first indicator of Mood changes, which is why I always ask my patients about their sleep and sleep patterns at every visit. Most new patients arrive with sleep symptoms. Most current and returning patients report sleep improvement as treatment of Depression progresses.

A number of new patients come in for a first visit, concerned about their changes in sleep. Many of them suspect at some deeper level that the sleep problem is probably serious, but they may not suspect Depression as the cause. But, they do suspect they have a serious problem—otherwise why would they come to see a psychiatrist—or be sent to see a psychiatrist? One reason is because their family doctor might have refused to give them any more sleeping pills, but that is not always the driving force behind first visits. A second reason may be that they started out with somatizing symptoms, that are getting worse and are now disrupting sleep, in which case their family doctor has also sent them. They may feel bad but may not yet be aware that they have Depression. Or, thirdly, their family doctor told them this diagnosis (Depression), which they refuse to believe: such patients come to the first visit, expecting a diagnosis of insomnia accompanied by a six-month supply of sleeping pills, which will almost never happen (in my office). A few first-time patients are aware of the Depression. And a few people have such a serious sleep disturbance, that they feel they need to see a specialist because of sleep symptoms —these people obviously have a serious sleep problem, if they are willing to start with a psychiatrist! Many people think that sleep is the primary diagnosis. They are not aware that Depression is the primary diagnosis, and that sleep problems are just symptoms of the Depression diagnosis.

When people become Depressed, sleep patterns can deteriorate in two ways: there can be a change in the quantity of hours slept or a change in quality of sleep. If quantity changes, patients have an actual number of hours to report: "I'm only sleeping five hours a night"; hence, this is like a sign of Depression because it can be measured numerically. In altered quality, patients have a general impression of bad sleep that is sometimes not easy for them to measure and not easy to describe; this is like a symptom, because it is something that the patient feels but the doctor cannot directly observe or measure—unless the patient spends the night in a Sleep Lab, which is not a necessary procedure for sleep changes related to Depression.

In the case of altered quantity, a big complaint is fewer hours asleep. Marc may be spending "hours" trying to go to sleep or he is awakening too early in the morning—either of these problems will result in a decrease in the amount of hours slept. And this makes Marc feel tired (not enough physical rest), frustrated (seeming loss of control over sleep cycles), and irritable (brain hormones did not replenish during the night and cortisol levels are off kilter). If he drops from eight-nine hours of nightly sleep to five-six hours, he may feel a little "jumpy" every morning and then too tired in the afternoon (due to being deprived of two normal hours of sleep). Too few hours asleep usually result in daytime fatigue, poor concentration, and limited attention span, which many people think is ADHD. On the other hand, a person may report sleeping for too many hours. Or he may sleep too much for some nights and too little on other nights—this erratic pattern will not—

unfortunately—balance out as if "too many" plus "too few" equals "just right." Quite the contrary, this situation of wildly alternating quantities of sleep-hours can be a real emotional roller coaster. If Barney usually sleeps eight hours each night and then starts sleeping nine-twelve hours, he may feel that he is wasting time, or he may feel a little "jumpy" every morning.

Other quantities that may be measured (in a sleep lab) are the type and length of REM sleep and SWS cycles at night. REM is Rapid Eye Movement and SWS is Slow Wave Sleep. We already know how Depression changes REM and SWS, and we already know that these both improve when the Depression improves. In Depression, the number of total minutes spent in REM all night and the total number of REM sleep episodes will both decrease abnormally. We can also measure the four stages of Slow Wave Sleep (SWS) which are also usually decreased and imbalanced in Depression. (REM sleep alternates with Slow Wave Sleep all night long). The true purpose of SWS and REM sleep is debated, but we do know that everyone needs to have normalized cycles of SWS and REM—otherwise he will feel bad. It is true that some people naturally need more sleep, and some need less (this is not discussed here but can be found in *Everyone's Everyday Guide to Practical Psychiatry*). We still know little about sleep disorders. As mentioned, Depressed patients do not routinely go to the sleep lab, as we know that Depression causes all these numerical changes in sleep cycle. In the rare case that the sleep is severely disrupted despite adequate Depression treatment, then the patient might go to a sleep lab for overnight observation.

In other cases, there may be a reduction in quality of sleep. Patients often report that their hours in bed are about the same, but they complain of more awakenings during the night (tossing and turning) and too many "weird dreams." Since most "normal" dreams seem weird, anyway, this weirdness is not the real problem. The real problem is not "weird dreams," but rather that patients have more *remembered* dreams. We all dream a few or several times each night, but it is only normal to remember the last dream of the morning before awakening. Remembering more of the dreams from all night suggests a poor sleep pattern. A really big complaint centers around symptoms suggesting that the person does not feel "restored" to mental well-being each morning; therefore, we call this "non-restorative sleep." Decrease in quality of sleep is a symptom of a developing psychiatric disorder that will probably worsen. At some point, the quality may deteriorate further as indicated by new onset of nightmares. Nightmares are not necessarily a part of Depression, but they may occur and increase in some types of Depression. As Depression progresses, patients develop sleep symptoms of both poor quality and abnormal quantity.

When a Depression is mild, there are fewer symptoms. If the Depression worsens or if the Depression is not treated, then the sleep symptoms will usually increase and worsen, also. Some people with mild Depression might have only a change in hours of sleep (sign), whereas other people with mild Depression might have only the symptoms of poor quality of sleep (tossing and turning). However, people with severe Depression usually have both signs and symptoms of poor sleep that may be further accompanied by dramatic changes in sleep: nightmares, pacing round the house all night, sleepwalking, episodes of sleep paralysis, and so on. What really matters is that signs and symptoms are distressing to patients: these changes in sleep pattern are a red flag that an underlying Depression may be present and may often be one of the main reasons that the patient is coming to see a psychiatrist.

After people agree to try an antidepressant, their sleep should improve after a couple weeks and then continue to improve week by week until the sleep pattern is as good as it was before the Depression—this overall improvement may take months. In some cases, sleep is "better than ever," suggesting that there had been a mild Depression percolating for a long time prior to diagnosis. After a Depression is successfully treated, sleep should once again be "restorative." It is wonderful to see how much better people feel with good sleep, and the degree of sleep improvement is always a good indicator of the improvement in the Depression. The reader might not be surprised to learn that sleep can improve with the use of antidepressants, but might be surprised to learn that any appropriate antidepressant will restore sleep. A stimulating antidepressant can work as well as a sedating antidepressant. Patients who take stimulating antidepressants in the daytime will stay awake all day and not nap, thus they will be able to sleep well at night. People who take sedating antidepressants at night will obviously sleep better because of sedation. Any kind of antidepressant is restorative as long as it is appropriate for that kind of Depression.

Sleep should definitely improve with treatment of the underlying Depression, unless the person is suffering from a real medical disorder, such as sleep apnea, restless legs, or other medical and neurological diseases.

Sleep apnea occurs commonly in overweight and obese people—its main symptom is excessive daytime sleepiness (EDS) and its main sign is serious nighttime snoring. The treatment for Sleep Apnea is not a pill, but rather a breathing machine (with or without throat surgery). A similar breathing problem may also occur in late-stage emphysema when the lungs are over-inflated. Restless Legs Syndrome (RLS) is a neurological disorder that is nowadays being recognized as a common source of sleep disturbance, especially in women and in persons who are taking certain medications, including some antidepressants. (See RLS in the antidepressant list in Part Three.) There are several other medical conditions that can disrupt quantity or quality of sleep, such as blood vessel disease and other neurologic conditions.

Many years ago, we reassured patients that "nobody dies from lack of sleep"; however, that belief is being challenged now. Perhaps, no one dies as a direct cause of sleeplessness (it is not inherently dangerous like very high blood pressure), but there may be deaths as an indirect cause (inattentiveness). Depressed insomniacs may try to drink liquor to go to sleep—or they may obtain addicting sleeping pills; both of these ploys will cause additional problems later and will not restore normal sleep. Alcohol and addicting sleeping pills mainly serve to cause further disruptions in already abnormal sleep cycles. Knocking yourself out every night is nor normal sleep. If you have a sleep disturbance, please get it diagnosed. Most sleep problems can be successfully treated, whether they are caused by medical, neurological, or psychiatric diseases. I believe that sleep is one of the most important symptoms to treat in Depression. Sleep well, feel well.

AVOIDANCE

This situation is not necessarily about sleeping or napping, but is about hiding in bed. In the early stages of a Depression, a nap can be restorative and helps "recharge" the brain. However, as the Depression wears on, there is no more "recharging," but the person will try to recharge anyway, since that ploy had worked well at the beginning of the Depression. However, as the Depression progresses, there is no more recharging and the person is just trying to avoid contact with the world. Avoidance is necessary because the person is now depleted of his "brain hormones" and has no energy, motivation, or spontaneity for dealing with other people. Long telephone calls and surprise visits can completely drain his mental reserves. It may take him hours to recharge after such an encounter. As his Depression worsens, he can no longer recharge, and then he will feel doubly frustrated with the unwanted intrusion plus his inability to recharge. The usual method of avoidance is by screening telephone calls and not answering the door: the person is not being rude; he is just trying to make it through one more day.

INTERESTS

Depressed people start to lose interest in their usual activities. The most physically demanding pastimes and most mentally taxing hobbies may be dropped first. The Depressive may stop playing soccer, give up volunteerism, or quit doing crossword puzzles. As the Depression proceeds, routine physical activities decrease. There is a loss of participation in arts, crafts, gardening, basic home and auto maintenance, housekeeping, cooking, and so on. People who love to eat may frequently mention loss of food appetite as their primary concern. The person may give up reading because he cannot focus or remember the written material. In severe Depression, there is a genuine loss of interest in everything. He may watch TV, but remembers none of it, or is left unmoved by the TV program. He might also burst into tears for no apparent reason while watching TV. He may stare at the TV trying to follow plots, then gives up, and goes to [hide in] bed.

EXISTENCE

As Depression progresses, a person may question the value of life. In moderate Depression, philosophical issues about life and death arise and are then replaced by a total lack of will to live. In severe Depression, he feels that life is hopeless and that he is trapped without exit. This is rarely true, but the Depression robs Depressives of good judgment and the ability to see the situation as it is—that it is merely a treatable

Depression and need not be the end of the world. Which leads to judgment issues.

JUDGMENT

Judgment may be compromised in mild Depression as a person casts about to try to finance some diversion that he believes will treat the symptoms of the Depression. This will not happen, and in moderate Depression, larger sums of money will be spent on cars, trucks, electronics goods in the hopes of self-treating a mood state with consumerism. Eventually, judgment deteriorates to the point that the value of life itself is questioned and often found lacking. Any thoughts of suicide are Depressive symptoms but the plans to carry out those plans reveal a serious deficiency in judgment.

INSIGHT

Insight is the ability to observe situations and to interpret them "correctly." (Obviously "correctness" may vary depending upon one's own circumstances, but we all have an idea of what that may or may not be.) In early Depression, there may be a lack of insight because Marc does not even realize that he is Depressed. If he is told and shown that he is Depressed, and he still refuses to admit it, he is having some serious insight problems—and is also in denial of the problem. Some Depressives may sink so far into a Depression, that they have abandoned all self-care and are at risk of letting themselves be medically compromised by not tending to mental health and physical health issues. These are cases showing a severe lack of insight. These people may be forced into a psychiatric hospital because their severe lack of insight is jeopardizing their health.

ENERGY

As Depression progresses, physical energy may seem to drain away. This may partly be on a nutritional basis, but is mainly on a nervous basis. The nutritional basis may occur due to a lack of nourishing food or due to an excess of junk-food. On a nervous basis, the brain sends electrochemical messages to the muscles to move. This message is sent down the nerves to the specific muscles. In this sense, the brain is like a computer mainframe that communicates with desktop monitors via phone wires. If the brain is browning out, it will stop sending out so many messages, and the message may be weak. With fewer electrochemical messages, the muscles receive fewer orders to move and react. As a result of the tired brain, Dolores is slow to act, think, and speak and when she does speak, there are only short unfinished phrases. As the Depression worsens, she slows even further and feels very fatigued.

MENTAL ACTIVITY (CONCENTRATION, ATTENTION, AND MEMORY)

Since Depression robs a person of energy, then he naturally has a decrease in mental energy and activities, such as concentration, attention, and memory. He enters a state of mild mental Depression in which his attention and concentration decrease. Some modern Americans will suddenly jump to the erroneous conclusion that they have ADHD, which is not true. If they succeed in convincing a doctor to treat them for ADHD, then they will receive antidepressants, anyway, because all the ADHD treatments are actually antidepressants. If the Depression improves, then they will take this as proof that their "ADHD" has improved with treatment. However, this is imperfect treatment of a Depression, basically an "under-treatment." If Depression is under-treated, then the treatment will be imperfect as will the outcome, potentially. An under-treated mild Depression usually continues as such, producing a condition in which a person feels half-better or less bad, but not great. In some cases, an under-treated mild Depression could become a moderate—or even—a severe Depression, at which time, mental concentration will become so poor that memory problems ensue. In severe Depression, Hilda may become confused also and not be able to think clearly: she may even deteriorate to the point of having psychotic symptoms at which point she is completely divorced from reality.

If a mild Depression is treated as ADHD (with amphetamines), it may suddenly seem to improve in the first couple days, but there will be a sudden lapse back into Depressive symptoms for a while. It will later improve, somewhat, but the treatment outcome may be suboptimal (dosage adjustments and maneuvers will not be performed as required in treatment of a Depression). If a mild Depression is treated as ADHD (with non-amphetamines), then it will follow a course of treatment similar to that of a true Depression that requires a few weeks to recover. But once again, dosage adjustments and other maneuvers may or may not take place. Sometimes in these misdiagnosed cases, the non-addicting ADHD medication will be raised sequentially several times, which mimics Depression treatment, and is often a dead give-away that a Depression is under treatment and not ADHD, even though the diagnosis of record is ADHD.

Typically, in the treatment of Depression, recovery is slow and gradual. Medication adjustments take place, and secondary medications may be added onto the primary antidepressant. A mild Depression may seem somewhat better for as long as the medications are continued. Moderate Depression is rarely confused with ADHD because it has more symptoms which are obviously Depressive in origin. Severe Depression has a host of serious symptoms (as listed here) and would not be confused with ADHD. After a severe Depression is successfully treated, patients may have only a hazy recall of all the details of their sickness. They may not easily remember exactly what had happened because their memories were so impaired and they were so confused. Patients with mild and moderate Depressions, however, can usually remember the course of the Depression and its treatment fairly well.

ACTIVATION

Depressives can also have episodes in which they become fretful, then anxious, and this can progress to agitation. There may be agitated outbursts interspersed with episodes of fatigue. These activation episodes might relate to sudden alterations in brain hormones. In severe psychotic Depressions, there might even be extreme excitement in which the person engages in rapid, repetitive, and purposeless activity that can last for hours and then be followed by an emotionless and motionless state (catatonia).

ISOLATION

Depressives usually tend to isolate themselves, called self-isolation. They have no interest in and no energy for dealing with other people. In the early stages of a mild Depression, they like to stay at home, but they may sense that this is abnormal, especially if they had had a typical social life previously. They may drag themselves out to do a minor errand or to window-shop. While they are out of the house briefly, they may feel detached from the world, as if in a dreamy state; they may forget why they left home, whereupon they return home, to their comfort zone, and resume solitary activities. They may fear bumping into acquaintances in public because they have no motivation to socialize—even superficially. They feel weak at home alone, but also feel safe and insulated. Perhaps a nap will be helpful, but they awaken with a sense that a chunk of time has been lost from their life and they do not feel lively or restored. This empty realization may neutralize any benefits from the nap. Depressives will often shun long excursions out of the house: they have little energy for walking around the mall or car show. They do not like crowds or long checkout lines because this forces them to spend more time out of their comfort zone (their home). They do not have a phobia about being in open spaces or some primary anxiety disorder—they just want to be at home. They do not have panic attacks in public, just distress over "wasting time." And yet, if they were home, they would still have some sense of wasting time, anyway. They may have an altered sense of time as if time were moving sometimes too quickly and then too slowly. There is a sense that the weekend has been "fast-forwarded" to Monday morning—time to go to work again and to try to appear productive. As a result of all these symptoms, they may choose to go shopping at odd hours in 24-hour supermarkets.

As Depression progresses to the moderate stage, they are likelier to shut themselves in the home. Then they have no interest in appearing in public, looking unkempt and feeling frayed. They may order take-out food to be delivered—when they have an appetite. They shut themselves up in their houses during moderate Depression. By the point of severe Depression, they shut themselves up in their rooms and their eating habits become bizarre or non-existent.

On rare occasions when they are coaxed out of their isolation cocoon and forced to socialize, they might drink too much in the hopes that it might make them sociable and chatty. This can have unexpected consequences in the case that they drink too much. Or they might actually put on appearances as a non-Depressed person for an hour or so, in which case, friends and family will think that their Depressive symptoms are under voluntary control and, hence, not valid symptoms. Based on this good showing, they will be expected to act just like non-Depressed people for the other twenty-three hours of the day. This will obviously not work out. Using alcohol to try to become someone else does not provide any real long-term benefit.

GRAY SHADE

In a mild Depression, the world still retains its color, but it is not so vivid or so noticeable as it once was—the patient may see the world as if it were a colorized black-and-white movie. As the Depression progresses, the world seems to lose color or look washed out, and eventually everything looks drab. The same may happen to music, also, which merely becomes a series of sounds, and then later, music becomes noise—or is not even perceived.

MOOD

Mood, of course, is affected since Depression is considered to be a Mood Disorder, although as the reader can see from all these listed symptoms, that Depression could just as easily have been called an activity disorder or a sleep disorder. Early in Depression, the mood becomes less "bouncy." There is a loss of desire to laugh. The person may appear saddened, although sadness is not the only mood change in Depression. There will be less bliss and less mirth. Meg or Hilda may retain the ability to put forth a "good face" for short time periods, but the effort leaves her exhausted afterwards, perhaps in need of a "restorative" nap; although, as the Depression deepens, naps will no longer be restorative, and instead will be just a time-out from society. As the Depression continues, she becomes gloomy and sees the glass as half empty, not half full. She may start to cry more readily over sad events, bad memories, and tragic movies. Alternatively, she may simply not have the energy to have any emotions. Other people will say that she is sulking or brooding, which is only a half-truth at best.

When she reaches the point of a severe Depression, she may be pessimistic, sad, and constantly unhappy and discontent. She may ruminate about all her past unhappinesses; the world is interpreted as doomed, gloomy, and devoid of goals and purpose. She will enter a state where she feels hopeless, helpless, hapless, and friendless. Life and death may be indistinguishable, in her opinion or from her viewpoint. This is how she arrives at the point of suicide. At this point, she may lack any mood except for one very dark, empty, and deeply Depressed mood, like a Black Hole of Depression. If she passes over the emotional "event horizon," then she may be lost—Depression needs to be recognized and treated long before arriving at this point.

LIBIDO

Libido refers to sexual desire and sexual appetite. As Depression deepens, libido decreases and then is progressively lost. Extremely Depressed people are less likely to have children. Men lose the drive and desire, and sometimes the capability to perform. Women lose desire and drive, and may also have significant Depression-associated menstrual changes that are not conducive to conception.

THOUGHTS

Depressed people will at first view the whole process of becoming Depressed as unjust and purposeless and wonder why it happens to them. Then they see themselves as purposeless, too. They experience a fall in self-esteem. As the Depression deepens, their thoughts become more depressed, then sometimes bizarre. In severe Depressions, people may feel unrealistic thoughts about themselves, such as guilt. Marianne Faithfull expresses these feelings in her song *Guilt: "I feel guilt, though I've done nothing wrong, I feel guilt..."* Depressed people will also report feeling useless and worthless. This is an example of a symptom that is a characteristic feeling of moderate or severe Depression, and is not a psychotic symptom. So, mild, moderate, and severe Depressions do not have catastrophically bad thought symptoms.

In severe Depression, however, thoughts can worsen to the point of becoming psychotic: this is a Psychotic Depression. Three common psychotic symptoms are delusions, illusions, and hallucinations. These symptoms never reach the magnitude or characteristic of severe psychotic disorders such as schizophrenia. Usually a Psychotic Depression may have only one or two psychotic symptoms, usually a delusion. In contrast, people with psychotic illnesses (schizophrenia) have thousands of possible delusions, some of which are permanent but can be temporarily suppressed with anti-psychotic medications. Delusions in Depression are usually temporary and much more limited in scope and extent and they usually clear up with treatment. There are a number of other possible psychotic symptoms, but they are not typically found to any significant degree in Depression.

Delusions are commonest in Psychotic Depression. Delusions are fixed false beliefs. Since delusions are false beliefs, this means that the guilt is false, also. Examples of guilty delusions are feeling guilty about events over which one has no control. Other types of Depressed delusions are beliefs that one has no money, no value, or that one no longer exists. In order to be a true delusion, a patient like Hilda must believe that the delusion is true, she cannot be argued out her belief, and she must be willing to act on it (or already has) to her own detriment. For Hilda, the delusion is a true and reality-based belief, whereas her family can see that it is a fixed false belief, and that her acting on it will cause damage to her health and well-being.

Illusions are psychotic symptoms in which Hilda might see or hear something real that is simple and harmless, but she twists it around to have a serious and dangerous meaning to her. She sees a parked car and thinks that the IRS is spying on her. She hears a car backfiring and thinks that the IRS agents are firing guns into her house. When she calls the police to report this as a "fact," then there will be consequences for her. She may be sanctioned for a false police report. This is one way in which an illusion might cause her damage.

Hallucinations are also psychotic symptoms, but do not occur significantly in Psychotic Depression. Hallucinations are diagnosed when Hilda imagines that she hears, sees, touches, tastes, or smells something that has no existence in reality. Hilda might see imaginary children playing in the backyard (briefly), may hear some indistinct whisperings or mutterings "coming from somewhere" or may hear someone calling out her name a couple times a day, "Hilda! Hilda!"

Typically, delusions are the only main psychotic symptoms in Psychotic Depression. Psychotic Depression occurs usually in the older age groups, and less commonly, in middle age.

MESSAGE

This sums up in one phrase what the Depressed person thinks:

Mild Depression: "I'm tired."

Moderate Depression: "I'm miserable."

Severe Depression: "I wish I were dead…"

Severe Psychotic Depression: "I am dead."

(Here are some other psychotic examples: "I am the only reason that my children did not turn out well," "My brain is rotten," "I am bankrupt.")

DEGREE OF DEPRESSION

The degree of severity of the Depression has much to do with successful treatment and good outcome. Usually, the best outcome obtains when a Depression has only a few mild symptoms that are diagnosed and treated early (except for some cases of Dysthymia). The worst outcome can usually be predicted if a person has a severe Depression with many severe symptoms that have a delayed diagnosis and delayed treatment. An intermediate outcome can be anticipated for cases of moderate Depressions:

A person with a *mild Depression* might have a few mild symptoms with perhaps one moderate symptom. Examples of mild symptoms are: loss of appetite, trouble falling asleep at night, taking more naps on the weekends, decreased interest in socializing, avoiding going out of the house, boredom, lack of motivation, loss of interest in usual hobbies, unreasonable fretfulness, and uneasy sensations that something alien is settling into one's emotional being;

A person with a *moderate Depression* might have all the mild symptoms or just a few of the moderate symptoms. Moderate symptoms could include the following: further appetite loss, noticeable weight loss, trouble falling asleep, awakening too early in the morning, poor quality of sleep, napping all weekend without feeling restored, minimal interest in hobbies or sex, decreased interest in children and family, anxiety, social withdrawal, and wondering what death would be like. Courtney might take a small overdose to see what death would be like, but without dying or trying to die. Meg may also try to avoid long phone conversations and may refuse to see people except for close friends or family and even at that, any visits with them become exhaustive within half an hour;

A *severe Depression* would have severe symptoms and a few moderate symptoms; and, a very severe Depression might have all the severe symptoms plus suicidal gestures and psychosis (Psychotic Depression). Severe symptoms can include dramatic weight loss, physical weakness, pacing around the house at night, self-isolation in bedroom, avoiding all social contact, sleeping all day, and thoughts of death. Even beyond severe, Hilda might develop psychotic Depressive symptoms such as fixed false beliefs about the world. She may take a small overdose of some pills or drink bleach. Suicide becomes a real threat in some of these cases; the suicide may be intentional or accidental: intentional suicide occurs when Courtney purposely takes an overdose in the hopes of dying and accidental overdose occurs when Hilda forgets how many pills she has already taken and takes an extra dose plus several extra pills in the mistaken belief that more pills will make her better sooner.

Patients with *Dysthymia* have a few mild symptoms that are usually chronic: the symptoms do not change much from year to year and do not usually progress. Under some circumstances, dysthymic patients may be prone to acquire a Major Depression on top of the original Dysthymia. This is then called a "Double Depression" and is treated as a Major Depression. This can happen with some regularity in dysthymia; Double Depression can morph into a Chronic Depression (this can occur because Dysthymia is already a mild chronic Depression).

Mild Depressive patients can take care of themselves. Moderately Depressed persons may need some outside help until they feel better: they may refuse to cook, wash bed sheets, or do errands. They will usually bathe. Severe Depression requires a lot of monitoring, and much of that monitoring may come from the family. In some cases, the patient might need to be in a psychiatric hospital, especially if feeling suicidal or unable to take care of himself (as demonstrated by not cooking, not bathing, not eating, not paying bills).

COMMON RISK FACTORS FOR DEPRESSION

"depression" refers to the concept of sadness used in everyday speech
"depressed" means "sad"
"Depression" refers to the formal diagnosis of clinical Depression
"Depressive" is the person who has Depression
"Depressed" means that the person has been diagnosed with clinical Depression

Besides the known causes of Depression, there are certain factors that might come together and contribute to the likelihood of developing into a Depression. These risk factors occur commonly in the general population and could put anyone at risk of developing a Depression.

CHARACTERISTIC RISK FACTORS

How do we know if a certain person will become Depressed—and if so, with which type of Depression? The Depression may depend on various factors that come together at a certain time in a certain person to create certain characteristics. For example, take a student named Dan who is a survivor of childhood leukemia (he was cured). His father is an alcoholic, his brother has ADHD, and his great grandfather had died young, possibly from suicide. He and his friends are traveling to a high school football game when the school bus crashes and Dan is the only survivor. He may be left temporarily partially paralyzed (like Ben), but may make a moderate recovery after a year of physical therapy. His risk of developing Depression depends on a combination of factors such as severity of injuries, degree of recovery from the injuries, medical illness, family history, emotional trauma, and circumstances (survivor guilt, in this case). Very importantly, we wonder how many family genes he has inherited from his father's side of the family. He has a lot of risk factors that very well might "push him over the edge" into Depression. And he may likely develop some form of Depression with or without PTSD, also. We can try to predict which Depression he might develop—if any. Nonetheless, he is at high risk, based on all his risk factors.

Now if we take a student named Bob who has none of these risk factors, who comes from a family without known psychiatric history, and who makes a full recovery after the bus accident, then we can "guesstimate" that Bob has little chance of developing any significant Depression. Bob might likely develop a Reactive Depression due to loss of his friends, but this is not permanent. And he might have survivor guilt which can be treated with talk therapy over time. If we look at one hundred accidents with boys like Dan, and a hundred with Bob's, we will see that the Dan's are likelier to develop Chronic Depression, alcohol abuse, and so on. This type of stress can also set off a major mood disorder if Dan carries Bipolar or alcoholic genes. Bob is much less likely to develop a major form of Depression than Dan. So, what's the big deal, anyway? Very simply, the hundred boys like Dan need to receive pro-active and long-term psychotherapy after the accident, because they are at high risk. And, prevention may be the best treatment for Dan in the sense that early and long-term therapy can identify early symptoms, which can then be treated earlier before Depression becomes severe. If Bob refuses to go to therapy, this would be less of a concern that Dan's refusal.

Certain general statistical principles can inform us about such outcomes, such as taking into account the five important risk factors of genetics, environmental stress, upbringing, previous psychiatric illness, and medical illness. Many of these risk factors are totally unavoidable, some are modifiable, and a rare few are preventable. Usually unavoidable risk factors are genetics, serious medical illness, previous psychiatric conditions, accidents, grief, pregnancy, and bad upbringing. In the case of upbringing, even if Child Protective Services places an abused child in a foster home, this placement is still an unavoidable risk factor for the child.

Some factors may be modifiable such as environment, lifestyle-induced medical illnesses, and upbringing—in the case that an intervention on behalf of a child can actually improve his welfare. The risk of Winter Depression can be modified (decreased) by moving

South. Rare cases where risk factors can be voided include alcoholism, for example (those who never drink, never become alcoholic). Since the types of Depressions vary, the presence of risks may vary, being partly environmental or from upbringing, with only moderate genetic contribution.

Some genetic risk factors probably cannot be modified or controlled in any way—these are "accidents waiting to happen." Certain types of Manic Depression are genetically inherited, and there is no current technology to stave them off. The only pro-active measures that can be taken by a person with this family history is to learn more about his family history and learn to recognize early symptoms of Manic Depression. This self-knowledge may or may not be helpful if he becomes manic, but at least he will have some forewarning of the event. Another type of risk factor is genetic in which almost every generation of the family has at least one member who is affected with some type of Depression or Depression-Equivalent Disorder, such as ADHD or compulsive disorders (gambling, alcoholism, and so on). Whether a family member will get Depression or any of these disorders is quite variable. On the other hand, some genetic risk factors may be modifiable, such as the genetics for alcoholism and alcoholic Depression. If a person such as Gilbert has a majority of alcoholic relatives as well as alcoholic parents and grandparents, then he should assume that he carries those same genes. We all know that a person cannot become alcoholic if he never touches alcohol. Likewise, a person can never develop Alcoholic Depression if he never drinks. Gilbert must determine that he will never taste alcohol and train himself to avoid it at all costs. In Gilbert's case, self-knowledge may be very helpful, and he can modify and stave off his genetic destiny due to forewarning and foreknowledge. Unfortunately, in many of these cases, families have not kept detailed medical facts about relatives, and even in cases where they have, the diagnoses are sometimes questionable. And, of course, people like Gilbert can be armed and forewarned with much knowledge, but are still drawn uncontrollably to alcohol as a moth to a flame.

Environmental risk factors may be environmental or from family upbringing. As far as environmental, there may have been a possible episode of poisoning, a childhood illness (case of Dr. T), social stress, a temporary lack of oxygen to the brain (near-drowning experiences), an accidental blow to the head ("our son was never quite the same after that"), and so on. In the case of risk factors from upbringing, psychiatrists sometimes see a blended family of full siblings, half-siblings, stepsiblings, and foster children, all of whom are reared in the same environment, and all of whom seem to develop similar Depressions but who have little or nothing in common genetically. This certainly makes a case for upbringing and/or environment as risk factors. Some of these risk factors may be modifiable and some, not.

A person who already has other illnesses may be at increased risk of Depression. Such types of risk factors are medical illnesses, neurological illnesses, and a few primary psychiatric disorders.

Medical illnesses and neurological disorders that serve as risk factors include all those listed under "Causes of Depression" at the beginning of Part One as well as many others. A number of patients report feeling Depressed upon learning that they are coming down with a serious incurable medical or neurological disorder. This is technically a Reactive Depression and could occur with any serious disorder.

Other psychiatric conditions that can cause Depression include those likewise listed at the beginning of Part One. These are disorders such as severe long-standing Anxiety Disorders, as well as compulsive anxiety disorders (alcoholism, overeating, Obsessive-Compulsive Disorder, and so on). Anyone who has a drug or alcohol problem has a higher risk of becoming Depressed. This includes cases where he is addicted to prescription drugs, also. (This does not include situations of Reactive Depressions, for example, if a driver's license is confiscated for a third DUI.) Previous Depression is a significant risk factor for becoming Depressed again. Some people with a first Depression will improve then have a second episode of Depression later in life. About two-thirds of first time Depressions might get Depressed again, some of which may become chronic Depression.

STRESS AS AN ENVIRONMENTAL RISK FACTOR FOR DEPRESSION

Stress is a significant risk factor for Depression. Stress is a general term for a collection of stress factors (stressors). Stressor is usually just one stress factor or one event. However, if the event is prolonged and generalized, then it is probably better described as stress. So, what is stress? I would define stress as 'any source of unpleasantness or any out-of-the-ordinary factor that forces us to muster up a response with mental energy', which usually means that we must consume valuable brain hormones dealing with something that we consider annoyingly unplanned or unnecessary—something that we would not normally choose to do. The summoning up of this mental energy can result in thoughts, speech, or action—but no matter which of the three, the brain must turn its attention from its focus of concentration onto this extraneous interruption. However we define it, stress can make everything worse. Stress can make life seem unpleasant and miserable. Any major changes in the people, events, and things in our surroundings, or inside our bodies, can induce stress.

We are daily exposed to external and internal stressors. External stressors refer to our jobs, social status, finances, physical trauma, and so on. Internal stressors include spiritual and emotional upheavals as well as medical illness and consumption of chemical substances. A healthy person usually has a system for dealing with stress (yoga, aerobics, hiking, hobbies, sports, and so on)—if not, then a person needs to devise such a back-up system for routine stress relief.

A very important group of environmental risk factors results in stress. These are often associated with adults, but can also occur in younger ages. In children, frequent changing of schools can be stressful. Being teased by bullies can be stressful, as can parental divorce. In adults, we all recognize the stress of jobs, money management, family relationships, and so on; and, these have childhood equivalents, too.

Some people end up in situations which can lead to other situations which in their turn can promote stress and then Depression. Or these situations can make a susceptible person develop the onset of his first Depression. The outcome of whether or not a person becomes Depressed in these situations, may be softened by his system for dealing with stress. Environmental stress that may aggravate an early Depression might be political, social, or linked to financial disaster. Political stress can take a terrible toll on a population, leaving the survivors with varying types of Depression and crippling Anxiety Disorders (PTSD). Political stress may result in shaky governments accompanied by personal financial stress.

There are also socio-economic risk factors for Depression. These risk factors do not cause Depression, but may leave a person susceptible to developing Depression: frequent job-related moves, job stress (constant low-grade harassment), financial distress (bankruptcy), divorce, serious family problems, multiple bereavements, and prolonged residence in a foreign country (especially if that country is recognized as a "hardship post"). These summed risk factors or minor stressors may find their analogy in a pneumonia. For example, a woman in good physical health gets a cold. On the next day, her boss wants her to fly to Prague (involving three plane changes). On one leg of the flight, she is seated in front of two sneezing children and a cigar smoker, and after flying non-stop for twenty-three hours, her taxi breaks down and she has to walk to the hotel in a downpour. If confronted with only one or two of these stressors, a healthy young woman might not become ill, but the sum of all these factors (called "kindling") conspire to give her pneumonia (in our case, Mild Depression). Humidity, little children, sneezing, cabin air pressure, inhalation of common airplane air, cold rain, time zone stress ("circadian rhythm" disruption), and sleep deprivation cause biochemical stress to cause possible pneumonia in the same way that several minor emotional stressors in rapid succession on top of each other can result in a mild Depression (see Betty's story). This is only an analogy but serves to highlight the effects of kindling in bringing about a first-time Depression.

People are also surprised to find out that there are two types of stress: "good" stress and "bad" stress. Examples of "good stress" would be a pleasing but out-of-the-ordinary event, such as earning a large bonus, receiving fame and accolades, and so on. Examples of "bad stress" would be job termination, serious traffic accident, divorce, and so on. We could also list a third category of "not-good, not-bad stress": divorce (from a drunken husband or promiscuous wife), job loss (from a miserable job that has caused high blood pressure and chronic insomnia), traffic accident (in which the injured fell in love with one of the first responders), and so on. Obviously, the terms "good" and "bad" are quite relative. "Good" to Republicans might be "bad" to Democrats, "good people" in Islam are possibly "bad people" to fundamentalist Christians, and vice versa. As Shakespeare said, "there is no good or bad, but that thinking makes it so". "When bad things happen to good people" obviously requires us to divide half the population into good, and half, into bad—which is certainly a subjective exercise and a matter of opinion. Besides these types of stress, we can also suffer "ancient" stress (being chased by coyotes while hiking or beaten on the street by gang members) or "modern" stress (rush hour commutes, backstabbing office politics, job layoffs). It can all be stressful. Life by its nature is stressful, whether we are living in a traditional society or a technological society. It may cause Depression. Thank goodness, modern society has developed medications available for treatment, if such is desired.

GRIEF

Bereavement and grief can be followed by depression, especially in elderly widows and widowers—they begin to feel intense loneliness, which can aggravate depression into a Depression. Family problems can also cause or aggravate Depression: divorce, dysfunctional families, and "difficult" in-laws. (See story of Enrique.)

Delay to Treatment (Time Untreated): This is the length of time that a Depression has remained untreated. Like any other chronic disorder, the longer that the Depression festers, the harder it will be to treat. This can be a risk factor for prolonging the amount of time needed for recovery.

INTRODUCTION
TO
TYPES OF DEPRESSION

How nice it would be to write about the "Kinds of Depression". Unfortunately, Depression is not kind, so I write about the types of Depression. Depression has been described and classified in many ways by many doctors over many centuries. Classifying the types of Depression is often complex because there are many types of Depression and many ways of classifying them that have appeared over the years. Every textbook of psychiatry has its way of approaching this complex issue. Here is a simple system that I am using in this book, and I present it in its most basic form:

- Reactive Depression
- Minor Depression
- Dysthymia
- Major Depression
- Cycling Depressions
- Other Depressions
- Secondary Depressions

These types of Depression will be discussed further in the following pages and Part Two. My wish is to present the types of Depression in a simple fashion that is easy to understand and yet still conforms to the standard system used by American psychiatrists. The reader may ask how I arrived at just these seven types of Depression. The easiest way, perhaps, is to explain that these above types of Depression are based on variables of severity, duration, treatability, and occurrence; we may also use causes and risk factors as a further way of defining the types of Depression. Causes were discussed earlier in Part One, and risk factors were just discussed. The remaining variables of severity, duration, treatability, and occurrence are presented below.

SEVERITY

Doctors often classify Depressed Mood into four degrees of severity: mild, moderate, severe, and very severe psychotic Depression. In general, mild cases have fewer symptoms, are "easier" to treat, and respond quickly to treatment in a predictable or reliable pattern. Severe cases may be hard to treat, may involve psychosis and suicidal thoughts, and may require many medications, as well as psychiatric hospitalization— perhaps even shock treatment. Moderate cases are intermediate between mild and severe cases. The determination of which degree of severity can sometimes seem arbitrary, but rest assured that treatment is based on you and your symptoms and not on some arbitrary rating system.

Mild Depression does not cause a permanent disability. This type of Depression is usually easy to treat, and a lot of these persons do not regularly come in to see a psychiatrist. Some people may obtain a prescription from the family doctor, buy herbs such as St. John's Wort, treat with talk therapy alone, or not treat at all. And some treat this with alcohol—having one or two cocktails every evening. These patients can be started on a mild antidepressant and should start to recover quickly. They might need a stress leave from work for two weeks, giving them time to adjust to any new medications. Even this stress leave is hardly necessary if starting on a mild antidepressant.

In general, mild cases do not necessarily need to see a psychiatrist, but all are welcome to come in for a psychiatric opinion. In a perfect world, everyone should be able to have access to a psychiatrist—including those with mild Depressions. After all, there is no way for you or the family doctor to know with certainty that it is a mild Depression until confirmed by a psychiatrist. In a number of these cases, the family doctor treats the patients who never see a psychiatrist. In other cases, the family doctor is on the right track, but the patients need some fine-tuning modifications and are sent to see me. I am perfectly happy to see these patients a few times to adjust their medicines, and then send them back to see the family doctor, who can continue to see them and give refills—once these cases are better, there is little for me to do, and I can focus on the severest patients. Many of these mild cases referred from the family doctor may choose to continue seeing the psychiatrist for prescriptions and will come in a couple-few times a year for refills of mild medications for a mild Depression that has been successfully treated. Fortunately, mild cases of Depression are the commonest.

The course and outcome of mild Depression is often straightforward: most cases will recover after a while on adequate doses of a mild medicine. Some of these will never have another episode and some will have a repeat episode in the future. Some patients will end up with a permanent Depression, a Chronic Depression. We lack the technology now to predict which course which patient will take. A few will morph out of the mild Depression into other problems such as panic attacks. This also is unfortunate.

As the degree of severity increases, so does the need for treatment. As the severity increases, all these treatment issues worsen and increase also: (1) severer cases will need more medications, perhaps two-three-four psychiatric medications each day; (2) severer cases will likely remain ill for years or decades; (3) severer cases will be likelier to have a long-term treating psychiatrist. Primary care doctors do not want to treat complicated psychiatric cases: picking up refills every six months from the family doctor will be highly unlikely.

Typical examples of mild Depression are Reactive Depression, Minor Depression, Dysthymia, and mild Major Depression. Moderate Depression would include Cyclothymia (one of the Cycling Depressions), moderate Major Depression, Chronic Depression, Bipolar Depression, and Recurrent Unipolar Depression (RUPD). Severe Depression includes Manic Depression, serious Bipolar Depression, and Severe Major Depression. The "Other Depressions" and "Secondary Depressions" are usually mild or mild-moderate in degree.

DURATION AND TREATABILITY

Duration refers to how long the Depression might last. Depression can be brief and last for only a few months in which case, it would usually be considered very mild. However, it can last for a year or two, which is typical of a mild or moderate Depression. It may last for a few to several years. And in some cases, it can last forever, which is called a Chronic Depression. The duration is not necessarily related to the severity. A brief Depression is usually mild, but it could be moderate. A Depression of intermediate length is usually moderate, but could be mild or severe. A longer lasting Depression can be mild, moderate, or severe, but is usually moderately severe. A chronic Depression can be rather mild as in the case of Dysthymia, but it can also be quite severe, such as a psychotic Depression (Hilda). It can also be intermediate, as in the case of Dolores. The longer a Depression lasts, the harder it is to treat, usually. Brief Depressions often clear up with low dose of a mild antidepressant. Longer-lasting Depressions usually require higher doses of an antidepressant, the use of powerful antidepressants, or may even require the use of two or more medications.

The duration is also related to **treatability**. A highly treatable Depression is easier to treat. A Depression that is harder to treat is relatively resistant to treatment, hence less treatable (we say "treatment-refractory"). When a person becomes ill with Depression, we believe that the inherent nature of the Depression is more or less pre-determined as mild, moderate, or severe. This is the same as the "flu": some people get a mild case of "flu" and take off only two days from work; others have a moderate case and take off two weeks; and still other people, have severe "flu" and are hospitalized (and might even die). These are apparent examples of the treatability factor of "flu"; there is no apparent medical evidence to suggest that everyone is destined to have only mild "flu," or that the person has done something to aggravate his flu into a severe case. Of course, it is possible for someone to aggravate a mild case of "flu" by running around in cold weather in damp clothes or underdressed. We tend to believe the same of Depression: the nature of the Depression is probably "pre-determined"; however, some people seem to aggravate a mild Depression into a moderate Depression or a moderate Depression into a severe Depression. Possible ways to aggravate a Depression include: not seeking prompt treatment, not receiving appropriate treatment, drinking alcohol to excess every night, and adding unnecessary stressors to life (buying luxury items, buying on credit, and overspending).

Some people, like Meg, get ill with a mild Depression that is treatable, whereas some people become ill with a mild Depression that is less treatable: there is usually no way to know which. In the case of a treatable mild Depression, early treatment with a low dose of SSRI antidepressant (Paxil, for example) may be all that is necessary for a good outcome, provided that the Depression is susceptible to Paxil; this example of Depression would be considered highly treatable. However, if Meg has a mild Depression that does not respond to Paxil, then the mild Depression might stay the same or get worse, and in either case, it will require higher doses of Paxil: it is less treatable. It may be a mild Depression that is resistant to Paxil, and perhaps the doctor should have started off with Effexor or another antidepressant, but unfortunately, there is no way for us to know about these susceptibilities, since no blood tests have been developed to allow us to know Depression-susceptibilities—unlike the treatment of infections where such lab tests are routinely available. In the treatment of infections, the family doctor can order blood tests that will show susceptibility to erythromycin but resistance to penicillin, for example, so he knows to start the patient on erythromycin and not on penicillin. Unfortunately, there is not yet any such reliable blood test for treating Depression, so the treatment is based on the doctor's "sixth sense." The doctor in this case can try low-dose Paxil, then high-dose Paxil, then Effexor, then Wellbutrin. Marc with the hard-to-treat mild Depression may end up doing really well on very low dose of Norpramin (30 mg a day). The fact that Marc feels restored on such a low-dose corroborates the initial diagnosis of mild Depression. Had the doctor only known to start on Norpramin, then treatment could have begun sooner—but there is no way yet to know this. Additionally, medications like Paxil are the standard starting medications for treatment of mild Depression—nowadays, Norpramin is third-line treatment (see Bartholomew). This is a good case of a mild Depression that seems less treatable.

If untreated, mild Depression, just like an infection or diabetes, could fester and worsen as time goes on. The longer there is in delay of targeted and appropriate treatment, then the worse the mild Depression can become. It could become less treatable because it has festered. It might also become less treatable by morphing into a moderate Depression. It can definitely become less treatable if Marc or Sasha have been self-treating with marijuana or alcohol. Alcohol will always worsen Depression, because alcohol Depresses the brain. So, in some cases, the duration of the Depression is related to drug-resistance, treatability, and self-treatment.

If Marc has a moderate or severe Depression, then it may be, by nature, less treatable because it is not mild. Patients like Marc who become ill with a moderate Depression can start out with the symptoms of a mild Depression, but the Depression will quickly and predictably worsen, because that is the nature of a moderate Depression. If Marc comes for early treatment, the doctor knows only that the symptoms are mild and may therefore start off with treatment for a mild Depression—and of course, this treatment will not be very helpful since we are in the presence of a moderate Depression. As a result, the symptoms of the moderate Depression quickly progress and outpace the mild treatment, Paxil, in this case. The Depression keeps on progressing one step ahead of the treatment, and the doctor is often playing a game of catch-up with the Depression, giving Marc the impression that the doctor is under-treating the Depression. That is why we doctors obsess over naming and identifying all the possible types of Depression: so that we can recognize any subtle symptoms that would identify a seemingly mild Depression as a more serious moderate Depression needing stronger treatment from the very beginning. As psychiatrists gain more experience (both in age and time), we learn to try to pre-select antidepressants that are appropriate for mild Depression but that can pre-empt a moderate Depression in its earliest stages, if such a clinical suspicion exists in the doctor's mind. This requires him to develop a certain "sixth sense" about these matters. I often approach this dilemma (is it a mild or a potentially mild-moderate Depression?) by routinely starting apparently mildly Depressed patients like Betty on a mild antidepressant (such as an SSRI or SSNRI) plus giving them permission to take Trazodone at bedtime as needed for sleep. If she comes back in a week or two taking moderate doses of the SSRI plus Trazodone every night, then we are probably in the presence of a mild-moderate Depression, and the appropriate treatment is "automatically" being taken by her based on tacit permission to self-treat her own symptoms (under some medical supervision). If she comes back to the second visit taking only a low-dose of the SSRI, then we are merely in the presence of a mild Depression. Without the availability of lab tests (such as those available for antibiotic susceptibility), this is the current state of art for treating Depression.

Treatability: is an important concept because it is directly related to suffering (see paragraph above). People with the most easily treatable Depressions will feel the best in the sense of having the least suffering. The best way to make a Depression as treatable as possible is to identify the Depression at its earliest appearance and treat it aggressively without making patients ill from medication side effects, and also to treat it appropriately so as to decrease its duration and severity.

Occurrence: Depression can occur once or twice or multiple times. It may appear once and never leave, thus becoming a Chronic Depression. Apart from these time factors, Depression may have timed patterns of appearance: it may occur unpredictably, cyclically, or predictably.

Unpredictable Depressions can appear suddenly, spontaneously, independently, or erratically.
Depression that occurs suddenly may likely have a cause, such as environmental stress—this can be likened to the Depressive equivalent of PTSD. The suddenness itself is usually unpredictable, like an "emotional accident." These are not common.

Depression that occurs spontaneously and unpredictably usually appears for no apparent reason and under no identifiable circumstance. Its onset is fairly obvious and not gradual. These are usually of unknown cause and are common.

Depression may also occur independently of any apparent stressors. A person may develop and then recover completely from a first-time episode of Major Depression. Years later, that person might develop a second episode of Major Depression that is independent of the first episode. Additionally, these episodes do not count as a Recurrent Unipolar Depression. This occurs commonly, also.

Then there are other cases in which a person has one episode of Major Depression and remains symptom-free for many years until he inexplicably develops another type of Depression, such as a Secondary Depression later in life (Depression due to Alzheimer's). These I call erratic Depressions. These are quite common.

*Cyclic Depression can appear unpredictably, but they will **predictably always come back** again in a next cycle—this is included in the very definition of Cycling Depression.* Depression may occur and come back in cycles. This is one of the Cycling Depressions. This happens classically with all the cycling mood disorders, which are: cyclothymia (Raj), recurrent unipolar Depression (Barney), bipolar Depression (Carrie-Beth), Manic Depression (Chet, Hank), and others.

Predictable Depression appears suddenly, specifically, periodically, or seasonally, in a known or knowable pattern of occurrence.
A Depression can appear suddenly, within the context that it had been expected for quite a while, so it is, in a sense, predictable. These are very rare cases. Men like Phil Spector or Andrew Luster probably knew that their actions could have grave consequences but they also thought that they would never be called to task for them, or that if they were, they could still avoid punishment. But when their verdicts were read, they probably had a major Reactive Depression as they had known they would.

Sometimes, Depression is predictable in that it will appear seasonally or periodically, or only in the presence of one specific stressor. Every time that that specific stressor is experienced, predictably a Reactive Depression will occur. Every time that a young woman has to move back in with her disabled alcoholic mother, the young woman gets Depressed. This can be characteristic of Reactive Depression. Of course, a series of separate episodes of Reactive Depression can accumulate and set off a Major Depression ("kindling effect"). This can happen also with Other Depressions and Secondary Depressions.

Depression can occur in response to certain timed cues, and every time that that cue happens, the Depression may follow. Depression is seasonal when it occurs every winter—or more rarely, every summer. This is Seasonal Depression. Sometimes Depression can occur periodically, such as after each baby is born. This is called post-partum Depression. A woman who experiences this once, will have it recur in following pregnancies—and in those cases, it can become worse and worse after each baby. If a woman has mild post-partum Depression with the first baby, then she may have a moderate case after the second baby, a severe case after the third baby and if she has more babies after this, the next episodes of post-partum Depression can be so severe as to result in a very severe psychotic post-partum Depression. Most of these women know this outcome. Or the progression may limit itself to a moderate Depression after each childbirth, and not progress so horribly. Most women who have this type of Depression do not continue to bear (many more) children.

So, if we make a list incorporating all these above variables, we can go further to generate an expanded list of fifteen types of Depression from the basic seven. These fifteen types are presented next at the beginning of Part Two.

PART TWO

Types of Depression Explained with Illustrative Case Studies of Fictional Patients

Terminology:

"depression" refers to the concept of sadness used in everyday speech
"depressed" means "sad"
"Depression" refers to the formal diagnosis of clinical Depression
"Depressive" refers to the person with Depression
"Depressed" means that the person has been diagnosed with clinical Depression

INTRODUCTIONS TO CASE STUDIES

Part Two introduces various cases of fictional and fictionalized patients with Depression. Starting from the original seven types of Depression in Part One, I have gone on to generate an expanded list of fifteen types* of Depression. The name of the person appears after the type of Depression that he suffers.

- Reactive Depression—Bart, Jesse, Matt, Daisy
- Minor Depression—Ben, Betty, Hamid**
- Dysthymia—Sarah, Tim, Louise**
- Major Depression:
- *Mild Major Depression—Kirk, Ida*
- *Moderate Major Depression—Ariana*
- *Severe Major Depression—Florence;*
- *Severe Major Depression with Melancholy—Phyllis*
- *Severe Major Depression with Psychosis ("Psychotic Depression")—Hilda*
- *Chronic Depression—Dolores*
- *Double Depression—Sarah, Geb*
- Cycling Depressions:
- *Bipolar Depression—Clairice, Carrie-Beth*
- *Bipolar Depression in Borderline Syndrome—Courtney*
- *Manic Depression—Chet, Hank*
- *Cyclothymia—Raj*
- *Recurrent Uni-Polar Depression—Barney*
- Other Depressions: *Winter Depression (Meg, Clairice), postpartum Depression (Janice, Cecile), and Prolonged Grief Depression (Enrique, Altagracia)*

- Secondary Depressions due to *Medical Illness (Eirene, Dr. T.), Drug Addiction (Jerrold), Alcoholism, (Rhonda, Gilbert, Alberto, Sasha)*
- Depression associated with Child Abuse (Tiffany, Marc-Evan, Jerrold)
- Mixed Depression (Meg, Aimée)
- Terminal Depression: Suicide (Derek, Seth, Jerrold, Matt)

*The exact process of creating this expansion is explained for the especially interested reader in great detail in Appendix One.
**these are cases who have tried several medications with varying success

Types of Depression Explained and then followed by Realistic Case Studies

If the name of the Depression has been updated by the APA,
then that contemporary APA name (of the diagnosis)
will appear in parentheses beneath the descriptive diagnosis
from our list.
Information on treatment is given in Part Three,
which can be read before or after reading Part Two.

Part Two consists essentially of fifteen Sections, each corresponding to one type of Depression, as outlined at the beginning of Part Two. Each Section discusses a particular type of Depression and explains it. Then there will be the introduction of some typical and some unusual cases of fictional or (fictionalized) persons who have that diagnosis.

Each case study begins by introducing a fictional (or fictionalized) patient, his description, and his situation. Then there will be psychiatric commentary, which is the discussion and explanation of what is happening to this person from the psychiatric viewpoint. After the discussion, there is a diagnosis. This is followed by treatment recommendations. Treatment can include any of the treatments listed in Part Three, including Rx which refers specifically to medication. "Outcome" gives a forecast for the person's future: what his short-term and long-term prospects are for a good life. (In Medicine, outcome is properly called "prognosis").

REACTIVE DEPRESSION:

(APA DIAGNOSIS: "ADJUSTMENT DISORDER WITH DEPRESSED MOOD")

Reactive Depression is often caused by stress, typically following an emotional crisis such as significant disappointments over job, career, or romance. A major job disappointment is reflected in the case of Jerry. Jerry could no longer pay his mortgage and lost his house, and his car was repossessed. A typical teenage stressor is presented in the cases of Bart, Matt, and Daisy, but they have catastrophic outcomes. Bart's and Matt's stories both serve to highlight the fact that cases in psychiatry—as in any other branch of Medicine—can have a wide range of possible outcomes, even in cases of supposedly minor disorders.

The astute reader might argue that Reactive Depression is due to some environmental factor, therefore it has a known cause and should be classified as a Secondary Depression. We consider it as a Primary Depression because we do not know *how* the stress factor biochemically causes the reaction. In the Secondary Depressions due to hormonal imbalance, alcohol, or multiple sclerosis, for example, we know enough about the biochemical mechanisms to classify these as Secondary Depressions. Here is a good example with diabetes. Diabetes causes high levels of blood sugar, and this biochemical change is not known to cause Depression (Secondary Depression); however, some people who receive a diabetes Diagnosis may have a negative reaction or even a Depressive reaction to the news of this Diagnosis. This is a Reactive Depression. High sugar levels are not known to cause Depression directly. I have seen a number of newly diagnosed diabetics with this type of Reactive

Depression. Some of them believe that the diabetes and the reactive Depression entitle them to be on permanent disability but Reactive Depression is not a psychiatric disability. (Read my previous two books for information on psychiatric disability.)

Reactive Depression is mild as far as the degree of mood Depression, and is quite minor as Depressions are concerned. There are only a few symptoms present in any Reactive Depression patient at any given time; the symptoms usually have a fairly obvious onset, usually clear up after a few months, and oftentimes may not even need medications. Or if medications are needed, then only small doses of mild medications are needed. In many cases of Reactive Depression, a social treatment such as talk therapy with a psychotherapist may be the only treatment that is needed. (Reactive Depression is similar to "*Situational Depression*"; both are now properly called "*Adjustment Disorder with Depressed Mood.*")

BARTHOLOMEW (BART)

Bart is a high school football star who developed anxiety attacks after his girlfriend got pregnant. He started to self-treat his anxiety with large amounts of beer on the weekends. And then he became sad and started withdrawing from social events, skipping school, and receiving low grades which resulted in his not being allowed to play football.

His health plan authorized him to see a young psychiatrist who diagnosed Depression. His parents did not want him to take Prozac due to their personal biases. They were leery also of other SSRI medications like Zoloft or Paxil because of a new government alert about using antidepressants in teenagers (see Black Box, end of Part Three). The psychiatrist convinced them to let Bart try Lexapro anyway (an otherwise approved treatment in his age group) which caused him to have sexual problems* (perhaps not such a bad thing in this case, but Bartholomew felt that this side effect was a deal-killer). Then Bart tried Wellbutrin that made him extremely nervous, as did Cymbalta. Trazodone is not an option in young men because it can cause prolonged painful erections (priapism); Serzone was eliminated from consideration also, because of risk of liver failure. His mother was a nurse who had been taking Tofranil for many years. She had anxiety, panic, and mild Depression for which Tofranil had been very beneficial. Her aunt also was doing well with Tofranil. Tofranil is also beneficial for anxiety, Depression,

ADHD, and obsessions. So Bart was started on low-dose Tofranil. He was even given a cardiac check-up to find out if his heart was functioning normally, an appropriate move for all patients taking such antidepressants—especially for athletes and teenage boys.

After four weeks on Tofranil, he felt somewhat better, and he exaggerated his wellness to his parents. Then his grades came back up. He was allowed to play football once more.

He had still not told his parents about the pregnancy. To make things worse, this had been a brief relationship with someone whom he would never consider marrying.

Bart was well maintained on low-dose Tofranil. He felt better, and stopped bingeing on beer on the weekends. His grades improved because his concentration improved on Tofranil. However, he was having allergies so his mother gave him some decongestants to take. Later that day he was running and collapsed to the ground. He was rushed to the hospital but could not be resuscitated. He had had a massive heart attack.

Discussion: Bart has probable stress reaction to the pregnancy leading to anxiety and secondary Depressive reactions, punctuated with a brief reaction of "self-treatment" by abusing alcohol. There is family history in that Bart's mother and aunt also had minor Depression and anxiety, which is why they were taking Imipramine on a long-term basis. This is a common finding in such families: the males drink, and the females take pills.

Bart developed Anxiety over the pregnancy and he also felt Depressed because he thought his whole future would be seriously changed due to the pregnancy. He decided to use alcohol which is a "downer" for the brain—it can cause Depression in the brain in various ways. Alcohol can also cause anxiety the next day when its sedating effects wear off. Tofranil is effective for anxiety, Depression, and compulsive behaviors (drinking), so it is a reasonable choice. Unfortunately, Tofranil has been associated with sudden death in active teenage boys. It is true that every year a few high school athletes drop dead from sudden heart failure, whether they are taking antidepressants or not. Adding Tofranil into the mix only serves to increase these odds. Additionally, in some cases, teenage boys are taking stimulating decongestants for some reason. The reason may be for hay fever or allergies—however, boys know that these drugs also increase stamina, endurance, and eagerness, facts which have not gone unperceived by those who are seeking to enhance their levels of performance. Mixing Tofranil with decongestants just increases the risk of a cardiac event, especially in the very rare but susceptible high school athlete.

Diagnosis: Reactive Depression (Adjustment Disorder with Anxiety and Depression)

Rx: Tofranil with fatal outcome.

Treatment and Outcome: One of the SSRI's would have been a better choice; however, the best treatment for (this type of) initial stress-anxiety would have been for the parents to take him to weekly appointments with a counselor specializing in adolescents (without medications, at least in the beginning of treatment).

---

*the sexual problem was inability to have orgasm, a common side effect of some antidepressants

MATT AND DAISY

Matt and Daisy had grown up together on the same street; although she had lived far enough west that she was in a separate school district, that still did not prevent them from referring to this geographic coincidence as compelling evidence of their destiny. They had actually bumped into each other a couple times in their teens, but had not met face to face. They did finally meet when they were both in Art School, where Matt was studying in the faculty of automotive design, and Daisy was studying in performance arts.

They had an immediate attraction and began a whirlwind romance based on common interests. They had both converted to Buddhism during high school, both preferred Chinese vegetarian food, and both owned all the CD's made by Chris Rea. After a year and a few months, they had a major falling-out about each other's annoying little quirks and bad habits, that seemed to multiply quickly. This led to a termination of the relationship. Simultaneous to and slightly preceding this break up, Matt had become very interested in one of the new transfer students, Carlotta. He was intrigued by her and thought about her constantly. Eventually, he had started meeting her surreptitiously at The Café where they were ostensibly studying for class, but were mainly studying each other. Inevitably, they started a relationship at the same time that Matt broke up with Daisy. Even though Daisy had wanted to break up, she really just wanted Matt to stop all his bad habits and accept hers. But she could not verbalize this because she thought that she was right. She also thought that something was wrong with Matt, perhaps another love interest, which really upset her. The reality was that a lot of the women in the school were attracted to Matt, but many of the male students thought Daisy was "too weird."

When Matt "officially" broke up with her and dished out the 'we should see other people' speech, she was furious. She grabbed a handful of her ADHD drugs and swilled them down with straight bourbon. Then she became incapacitated and decided to write a suicide note to punish Matt after which she also took a number of aspirin and Benadryl pills. She really did not think that this would kill her, but she grew afraid that it might, so she recanted and went downstairs to tell her mother what she had done. She was so intoxicated, however, that she fell down the stairs and blacked out, perhaps not in order, though—her recall of that evening was very hazy. At any rate, her parents heard her fall at the foot of the stairs, found the suicide note, and called EMS who took her to the nearest ER where her stomach was pumped. When Matt was told of this, he was surprised but remained impassive because he was so besotted with Carlotta. Daisy, of course, survived the overdose, and she was then changed to a less dangerous ADHD medication.

In the meantime, Matt was completely enthralled with Carlotta, who, it turned out, was from a very wealthy family in Europe. The two of them spent Christmas there, and Matt was obsessed with Carlotta. The day after Christmas, however, Carlotta's mother had a mild heart attack, so Carlotta did not return to LA with Matt. Then he started to obsess about her, what she was doing, what she was saying in any of her three languages of fluency, and so on. Carlotta did take a leave of absence, and when she returned to school, she seemed to have changed so much, that Matt felt he hardly knew her. She had come back to Art School to collect her belongings and say goodbye because she was transferring to a university on the East Coast in order to live with Henri-Louis, her former fiancé, whom her parents had insisted that she marry.

When Matt heard this, he turned as white as a sheet and became frantic, imploring her to change her mind. He came to learn that she had had a long history with her fiancé, and although it was an on-again off-again relationship, it was definitely on-again. She murmured to Matt that he was a nice young man and would certainly have his pick of many of the female art students. Such exclamations as 'But I don't want them—I want you, Carlotta!' fell on deaf ears. Carlotta closed the door of her dorm room and told Matt to go to his. He was in such anguish and such turmoil, that he could not think. He felt absolutely insane. He decided to prove his love to Carlotta and took half a bottle of extra-strength Tylenol. Early the next morning, Matt's roommate found this note:

'Carlotta, I love you so much, I would die for you! I am ready to die for you! Come back to me! I love you more than life itself!'

An ambulance took Matt to the hospital. He was slightly groggy but coherent. After having his stomach pumped (several hours too late), he then told the doctors of the Tylenol, a gesture with which he had hoped to manipulate Carlotta's actions and feelings for him: she knew nothing of this and was already en route to the airport. In the meantime, Matt was given the antidote for Tylenol poisoning, Mucomyst, and the staff psychiatrist was called to the ER where Matt indicated that he did not want to die, just to get Carlotta's attention. Unfortunately, it was too late for the antidote, and Matt slowly succumbed to massive fatal liver destruction over the next three days while doctors and concerned friends and family members looked on and tried to comfort Matt, who was extremely upset about his impending death. Daisy did try to spend as much of that time with him as was permitted.

Discussion: very young people can be very impulsive. These types of mild gestures are not uncommonly seen in the ER. The large majority of "adventuristic" overdosers do survive, partly due to the fact that most of the highly dangerous sedatives and sleeping pills of yesteryear have been replaced with safer alternatives. Also, in many cases, these people want to make a dramatic gesture instead of really dying. The suicide gesture is a cry for help or an attention-seeking maneuver. A small handful of aspirin may cause stomach bleeding and other serious medical problems, but is not routinely fatal. ADHD drugs can cause sudden heart problems, but Daisy apparently took too few. What most people do not realize, however, is that Tylenol—even in smaller doses—can cause life-threatening progressive liver failure that slowly evolves over two or three days. The antidote, Mucomyst, must be given without delay, otherwise death is almost certain. If the antidote is given too late, then the liver will fail. Two to three days is not enough time to arrange for a liver transplant. Mental health providers have been trained to understand these types of cases, and we will be glad to see them on an emergent or urgent basis.

Females account for many of the pill and drug overdoses, and some may make this gesture more than once. Most survive, because the overdose is a gesturing cry for help. Females, who really want to die from an overdose, are likelier to succeed than those who are gesturing. In a sense, many men also gesture with drug overdoses, but the drug in those cases is often alcohol with or without street drugs (alcohol poisoning, in other words); additionally, the men do not formally acknowledge it as a suicide gesture, since that looks too "emotional." They just drink obscenely large amounts of alcohol. The alcohol/drug overdose may also have been done in a blackout or have caused a blackout, so that the man's memory about the details is sketchy. Obviously, men in these cases do not leave a suicide note—usually notes are only written when men are gesturing (like Matt) or when the man's chosen method of suicide seems obviously fatal: car crash, hanging, gunshot, and jumping. (However, there are people who do survive violent and usually fatal methods.) See more under the discussion about Suicide at the end of Part Two.

I have included the cases of Matt and Daisy under Minor Depression, because they had no intention of dying. They were reacting to being jilted. These cases show how different the outcome may be. Daisy took more pills than Matt and she took pills that would be considered more dangerous than Tylenol. She survived, but Matt died accidentally from taking a half bottle of an OTC medication that most people consider harmless. Some people might be able to survive a large Tylenol overdose and some may not.

Diagnosis: Reactive Depression, in both cases

Treatment: emergency treatment depending upon the type of overdose

Outcome: usually non-lethal except in certain cases (any other details on successfully overdosing are intentionally omitted) BEWARE!

All medications are poisons taken in small amounts—whether they are Rx, addicting, non-addicting, or OTC.

JESSE

Jesse worked very hard at his mid-level management job for several years. He worked from home on the weekdays and went to the office frequently on the weekends. The one major indulgence that he allowed himself was to bring his dog to the office on weekends. He was in line to be promoted to supervisor and seemed to be in first place as far as anyone in the office could tell. When he was passed over for this opportunity, losing to some outsider, he took it hard, but tried not to let anyone see his achingly sad feelings. So, he decided to stop overworking himself and to start enjoying himself. He cut back to a forty-five hour workweek, after which the newly-hired supervisor thought that Jesse was only going through the motions and laid him off. Jesse could no longer pay his mortgage and lost his house. His car was repossessed. His colleague Joan recognized that Jesse was sad after losing his possible promotion. She encouraged him to see a therapist who was able to have Jesse talk about his feelings. His therapist urged him to obtain a prescription from his family doctor (Zoloft). Later, his new supervisor did ask Jesse to come back to work part-time. He did continue working there until he found a much better job at a competing enterprise.

Diagnosis: Reactive Depression

Treatment: twelve sessions of talk therapy and optional low-dose Zoloft

Outcome: very good

MINOR DEPRESSION

(APA DIAGNOSIS: "DEPRESSION NOT OTHERWISE SPECIFIED")

Minor Depression is characterized by only a few mild symptoms and needs only minor treatment, such as psychotherapy with/without mild medications. Minor Depression is sometimes never seen by a psychiatrist and can be treated by the family doctor who often is the only treatment source (using 10 mg of Lexapro or 25-50 mg of Zoloft, for example). People with good insurance are likelier to see a psychiatrist. Or the patient may not even see any doctors and may start herself on St. John's Wort and join a support group or begin talk therapy with a psychologist or psychotherapist without any need (at that time) to see a psychiatrist for prescriptions. Minor Depression is a term based on the analogy to Major Depression and represents "lesser" and more manageable types of Depressions. Minor Depression, however, is a more "complete" Depression than mere Reactive Depression. Minor Depressions may sometimes be treatable with talk therapy or group therapy without need of medications, although most Americans will want to try a mild antidepressant in these case—not because it is medically necessary, but because that is our cultural philosophy. Most people want pills because they want to feel better instantly (probably because our modern society demands that we all feel better instantly). Regardless of treatment method, when Minor Depression is treated adequately, then Ben and Betty will have a better chance at full recovery. Unlike Reactive Depression, if Minor Depression is left untreated, the Minor Depression will follow one of three paths: it may well improve and go away on its own (like Reactive Depression); it may become "socked in" as a persistent Minor Depression; or, it may actually worsen and become a Major Depression.

Sometimes Minor Depression will drag on without relief, proving itself to be a nagging daily annoyance—such as in the cases of people who are married to a practicing alcoholic: as long as the alcoholic continues to drink, then the spouse will feel miserable (this might technically be a case of Dysthymia or "Secondary Depression"). In other cases, the Minor Depression can aggravate into a full-fledged Major Depression. It can be aggravated by a worsening of the original problem or by the addition of new factors that would make most people depressed. (Minor Depression is now properly called *Depression Not Otherwise Specified*)

BEN

Ben had had a normal American boyhood until age seventeen when he had a swimming pool accident on the high dive that left him partially paralyzed from the waist down. He had to give up all his usual activities and finished high school with much difficulty on crutches and at times in a wheelchair. He had not yet become depressed by the whole situation, but he soon would be when he saw most of his friends leave and go off to college. He had abandonment issues, loneliness, and no prospects for dating the girls in his peer group. Ben was referred into a support group where he met a young man named Fred, who was paralyzed from the waist down.

Ben did have the good fortune to be living in the suburbs near Wright State University, one of the first universities ever designed from the ground up (literally) as a totally handicapped-accessible and user-friendly university. He did attend WSU and earned a bachelor's degree in chemistry. He later got a job at a local corporation and put his new skills to good use. After a couple years, he went back and earned a masters degree, also. Ben was no longer living at home, but was only a couple miles from his family. By this time, he had a good job, a condo, and a specially outfitted car. He had thought he was doing well until he realized that he was ready to nestle down but he did not even have a girlfriend.

He felt sad and depressed and began to spend more time with his acquaintance, Fred, who by this time was drinking a lot of beer on the weekends. Ben did not like drinking that much but was able to connect with Fred about their apparently bleak future.

Then Ben became Depressed and felt sad every night. He could not sleep well, he tossed and turned at night, and he had unhappy dreams of the diving accident. He started to cry one night when watching the local news. He started to have trouble concentrating at work. He thought that something was wrong and after a few weeks of symptoms, he made an appointment with his family doctor. Both his family doctor and the EAP (Employees' Assistance Program) suggested that he see a psychiatrist, which he did. In the meantime, Fred had found a socially marginalized girlfriend of spotty moral standards with a full-blown alcohol and drug problem. She moved in with Fred. She and Fred fed into each other's addictions and they both became heavy daily drinkers. Their unpredictable behaviors made Ben more Depressed, so Ben began to avoid them.

In the meantime, Ben got busy and got better. He went back to support group besides joining a men's group at church. He took Trazodone, which was very helpful (the sexual side effect of Trazodone was not a significant issue in Ben's case). He met an older woman who liked him and who disliked sex, and they had an adequate relationship. She had his child thanks to modern medicine, and they later decided to become foster parents. They both felt pleased in that their life together was much better than it would have been if single. Meanwhile, Fred and his girlfriend died from driving drunk.

Discussion: young men with this type of story can have a range of emotional responses ranging from alcohol abuse to Reactive Depression, Minor Depression, Major Depression or even full-blown alcoholism and drug-addiction. Some young men will not develop any psychiatric response at all. I have chosen Minor Depression for Ben as an "intermediate" response. Some people are given lemons and can sense nothing but sourness; other people determine to make lemonade with these lemons. The ability to do this depends upon personal motivation and upbringing. Some people are constitutionally incapable of figuring out how to "make lemonade," and this is not their fault. It may be their shortcoming, but it is not their fault. It is no more their fault than being born with any other incapacity. Some people have acquired this ability by luck or skill or by imprinting on their parents' problem-solving techniques and ways of looking at life. Ben also had support from friends, family, the swim team, teachers, and church youth group. Fred had none of these advantages and somehow perished.

Diagnosis: Minor Depression

Treatment: continue groups and Trazodone.

Outcome: good. Ben will, however, get a Major Depression if he lives long enough (and if he survives bladder infections and other medical problems). This case also shows that some people are relatively resilient to situations that would Depress many people.

BETTY

Betty is twenty-seven years old and works in downtown Los Angeles as a paralegal at a high-powered law firm. She likes the firm and her job. She enjoys the challenges of the cases and also gets some vicarious thrills from being involved in a few famous cases and celebrity lawsuits. She is considering applying to law school. Betty works fifty to sixty hours a week, occasionally goes downtown to work on weekends, and makes herself available by cell phone to her supervising Partner. Her career seems to be going well, and she is happy.

And then within the space of a month she experiences some minor upsets to her otherwise well-controlled routine. First, she receives a notice from the IRS that they have rechecked her last tax return and have determined that she owes them over four hundred dollars in taxes and interest. She has always prided herself on managing money: she has taken care to have no credit card debt, she lives in a small condo, she takes the Gold Line/subway to work, and drives an economy car, leaving her with a small car payment and mortgage. This IRS issue is an annoyance that she turns over to an accountant. Then her grandfather has a "mini-stroke" in San Luis Obispo (SLO) and she takes off a few days work, with the result that she gets behind in some of her paperwork. By the time she drives up to SLO, he has recovered and she wonders if she should have waited for further status reports on his condition. She gets behind in her paperwork for three days and needs to come into the office for a weekend marathon of paperwork. Additionally, she has recently started dating a "nice guy" whom she thought she really liked, but he calls to cancel their next date and to tell her that he plans to get engaged to his prior girlfriend. And then her brother-in-law's brother is seriously wounded in Iraq. Any of these events by themselves would have been manageable to her, but for some reason she seems to spool down from the combination of them all.

She suddenly starts to have migraines, which she had never had in her life. After doing "research" on the Internet she mistakes the migraines for Multiple Sclerosis or a brain tumor and insists that her family doctor send her to a neurologist. Her accountant deals with the IRS, and they actually owe her twenty dollars. Her grandfather makes a full recovery, and her grandparents drive down to L.A. to visit for a day; she uses the tax refund to take them out to lunch at a famous diner in downtown LA. She meets another nice guy in the elevator, but feels cautious and reserved about him. The wounded veteran is transferred to the V.A. in Westwood and he is eligible for permanent disability payments, after waging a lengthy battle to secure his benefits. Despite these better-than-expected outcomes, Betty begins to feel less "sparkly" and is more interested in staying in her condo every weekend watching TV and napping with her cats. She goes down to the pool and sees the other nice guy again and he seems interested and available. She notices how handsome and athletic he is. She agrees to go out for a matinée and coffee. He turns out to be a struggling actor, part-time graphic artist, and lifeguard. She goes out with him, but feels sluggish and preoccupied with something in the back of her mind. A second date seems to be somewhat unlikely. Then she starts to sleep too much at night and on the weekends.

Betty calls one of her friends, Naomi, who is a social worker and they have lunch. Betty wants to talk and talk about her problems and feels that Naomi can really understand her well. Naomi wisely refers Betty to a therapist who later refers Betty to a psychiatrist who in turn gives Betty low-dose Prozac that does make her feel better.

Discussion: Betty has a minor Depression. This is probably a temporary Depression. This demonstrates the "kindling effect" of having a number of minor stressors convene at the same time and "send someone close to the edge (but not over the edge)" (see Risk Factors in Part One).

Diagnosis: Minor Depression.

Rx: Prozac worked well for her without interfering very much in her personal life: it caused a decrease in sexual desire sometimes, and other times created a heightened effect.

Outcome: is very good; She did start dating the lifeguard. She was accepted to a local law school. Her Depression resolved within several months and she stopped taking Prozac then, also. She did suddenly start to have panic attacks about ten years later and was wise enough to seek psychiatric help—with the encouragement of her husband, the working actor; those attacks cleared up within a year while on Zoloft; after this, she might never have a recurrence of any Depression or other psychiatric conditions.

HAMID

He has come to L.A. to learn English and Spanish. He misses his family and friends in Syria. He began to feel isolated despite being in class all day with other people. He became aware that he had lost interest in his chosen field of endeavor, that his grades were slipping, and that he did feel Depressed. He sought counseling at the University health center where it was decided to start him on Effexor. He responded well within a couple of weeks and seemed to be doing better. And then after a few weeks he felt as if he was relapsing back into his same depressive symptoms. The Effexor dose was increased twice and then he felt much better but developed a very annoying sexual problem (lack of orgasm). Since he was not in a relationship, this was not a big issue. Then he felt new-onset symptoms, which were side effects of high-dose Effexor. He felt antsy, tired, bloated and had headaches. The Effexor was lowered and Vivactil, added, at which time he felt good (this combination has been called 'California rocket fuel').

He continued this treatment for a year with adequate success, but then his student psychiatrist graduated, and Hamid was assigned a new "student" doctor who promptly discontinued the Vivactil, labeling it as an "old" drug. The Effexor was changed to Pristiq and Hamid felt as if he were in a transitional phase in which he was neither good nor bad. The new doctor would not change the dosage and told him that he will be fine, "Come back in three months."

Hamid requested a new doctor who tried to get a better response from his one medication. So, the third psychiatric resident doctor changed

Hamid to Remeron at which time he felt as if he were in an experiment. He gained twenty pounds on Remeron, felt tranquilized, and was huffy when playing recreational soccer. So then he was prescribed Norpramin in low dose which was slowly increased to the point that the target symptoms were 85% controlled and there was no one predominant side effect that was a deal-killer. Hamid had little sexual problem, good concentration, motivation, and minimal weight gain.

Discussion: This is not an unusual case. It highlights the differences in treatments that different psychiatrists will prescribe as an extension of their personal philosophies (plus these are still student doctors working loosely under the supervision of a University psychiatrist). Hamid has a minor Depression (or mild Major Depression) that responds well to usual medications. The second student doctor seems insensitive—the basis for his decision is unknown. He may have been influenced by a recent free dinner at a four-star restaurant compliments of the pharmaceutical industry. And he is still learning about pharmacology. Hamid finished his degree and went back to his country to work in international import/export. He will always retain a slight proclivity to become Depressed, but Depression will not recur until he becomes elderly.

Diagnosis: Minor Depression

Outcome: Good. The mild Depression responds well to a low dose of one standard medication. He will have a second moderate Depression later in life.

DYSTHYMIA

(CYCLOTHYMIA IS NOT LISTED HERE, BUT INSTEAD IS LISTED AMONG THE CYCLING DEPRESSIONS BENEATH MANIC DEPRESSION)

Dysthymia is a long-lasting / lifelong type of minor Depression. It has also been described as a mild chronic Depressive personality style, which is an excellent way to view it. It comes in three "flavors": a person can be born with it, in which case it is essentially a permanent personality trait. In the second flavor, a person acquires it around puberty or by early adulthood. There is a third flavor in which the dysthymia alternates cyclically, which is called Cyclothymia. Regardless of "flavor," all Dysthymic people tend to be cynical, less motivated, and even pessimistic at times; they often try hard to mask or control the dysthymia—but usually without success.

Dysthymia is characterized by mild Depressive symptoms that are not disabling, but may reduce a person's efficiency to about 70%. Quality of life could be expected likewise to be reduced by about 30%. Dysthymia does not need to be treated, but life is much better if it is. Nowadays it can be easily treated with a mild antidepressant. Since it never changes its nature, there is little need to change antidepressants once a good one is found. This same antidepressant may be taken for years, unless the person starts to develop "resistance" to its effects, in which case it can be changed to another mild antidepressant. Dysthymia can also be treated with psychotherapy alone, but the treatment would need to be on a weekly basis indefinitely since dysthymia lasts indefinitely—unless a second condition is added to the dysthymia, such as Major Depression, at which point the combination of Depressions would best be treated with medication (see Double Depression under the Section on Major Depression). Additionally, and unfortunately, weekly therapy can be pricier than antidepressants. Apart from all that, dysthymia is a chronic mild Depression, sometimes referred to as a Depressive personality (in psychiatry, a personality style is permanent throughout the whole life of the person). The risk of suicide from Dysthymia alone is low; the risk may be higher if the person acquires a second major diagnosis such as alcohol abuse, panic attacks, or Major Depression.

SARAH

Sarah had always been a quiet, shy, and withdrawn little girl since she was a baby. She had few friends in school and focused mainly on hobbies such as gardening, pie-making, and collecting gemstones plus costume jewelry. Her parents did take her to see a child psychiatrist when she was around twelve, and she was diagnosed with Dysthymia, which her parents declined to treat with medications until she was a teenager at which time they would let her make her own decision. Finally, she did opt for a trial of very low-dose Prozac at 5 mg (at that time the only SSRI approved for use in teenagers).

With the new medication, she could concentrate better on homework and became less timid, but it did not change her overall personality. Her only boyfriend, Bob, was in the Science Club in high school, and they had a very slowly evolving relationship. They seemed well matched.

She went off to college and met Justin who was the opposite of herself and Bob. Justin and Sarah had a whirlwind relationship punctuated by passionate afternoon meetings between classes. He was a flamboyant and charismatic daredevil upperclassman. She was completely overcome by this relationship, which was something that she had never even imagined as possible before. Indeed, she was in limerence, although she did not yet know that word (the intense state of early passionate obsession in a serious romance). She had assumed that movies exaggerated the possibilities. Or that these were affairs that would never happen to her, as previously unimagined by her. Justin became the sole focus in her life and she was enthralled by his affection, attention, charisma, and gregariousness.

Tragically, he was taken from her by a fatal motorcycle accident. She went into such deep mourning that she had never known and vowed to wear black for the rest of her life. Her feelings were not altered in any way by the viewing, the funeral, or the dinner at which she began to piece together more facts about this man of her dreams. He had several ex-girlfriends, another current girlfriend, a serious drug addiction, and massive debts. These facts did nothing to soften her Depression and only made it more painful and deeply rooted as she turned to counseling for answers.

In counseling, she began to understand what had happened and was also able to put it into focus, viewing it through the lens of her family history of Depression and alcoholism. (She had not previously realized that she had a few relatives who were functional alcoholics.) Nonetheless, she did not feel better, and was absolutely certain that all chances for happiness were gone. Her Prozac dosage was increased twice with little benefit so bedtime Trazodone was added. She began to sleep better and feel better. She was also sent to a few Alanon meetings, but dropped out.

After all this, she met an engineering graduate student with whom she began to share a relationship. She was now realistically paired with someone whom she later married. She still took moderate dose Prozac and low-dose Trazodone at bedtime, and her symptoms were all controlled. She had tried to quit the medications, but felt worse without them.

After her first baby, she began to feel Depressed again as if the medications were not helping. She saw a new psychiatrist who adjusted her Prozac and Trazodone a few times, but she seemed to be no better. Her husband went to the next appointment with her and gave valuable information to the psychiatrist who then added a third medication, a mood stabilizer which brought her into focus within a week, and after a month she was feeling great despite having some minor side effects.

Discussion and Diagnosis: Sarah has had a Dysthymia all her life. Then she had a grief reaction that bloated into a mild Major Depression. And then she had a Postpartum Depression. She has experienced three types of Depression, at least two of them simultaneously. Besides medications, she also needs to have some therapy sessions from time to time. People with a pre-existing Depression (Dysthymia) are more susceptible to acquiring other types of Depression. She also has some family genetic traits in the form of alcoholism that favor Depression (alcoholism is a Depression-equivalent disorder—see Risk Factors in Part One).

Treatment: Medications will likely be needed for a long time, also. Alanon may still be helpful if she chooses to attend any type of group therapy.

Outcome: fair to good as long as she continues in regular therapy sessions for several years to come. This case serves to highlight the fact that people with dysthymia are more prone to develop other forms of Depression, such as Grief, Other Depressions, and Major Depression— the combination of dysthymia and Major Depression is called "Double Depression."

TIM

(Tim is elder brother to Aimée and Marc-Evan.)

Tim was an excellent and popular student in high school, a "red-blooded" American boy. He excelled academically and athletically. He was on the baseball team and was consistently on the honor roll. He had other athletic pursuits and had been voted MVP. He was the salutatorian of his graduating high school class, and had received a partial scholarship to Famous University.

However, Tim had one weakness and one flaw. His flaw was the love of gambling. His weakness was that he had famously bad judgment about girlfriends and women. He based his whole relationship with females on how beautiful they were and how much they inflated his ego. A beautiful girlfriend who doted on Tim could get him to do almost anything (legal).

When he had been in high school, he started to date Rhonda in his junior year because she was beautiful. She constantly told him how handsome he was and was always available for his every whim (except when she was passed out on cough syrup or her mother's pills). She was also sexually available and they had a brief but torrid relationship, which was why it was so hard for Tim to break up with her. All his teammates told him that she was a "closet alcoholic" and urged him to drop her. On their fifth date he went with his teammate, Tom, to pick her up for a double date; she swung the door wide open and was standing there wearing only satin underwear, talking rapidly, and she had blood running down from one nostril. Tim told her that he would come back in an hour, but did not do so, and he moved on to other pursuits.

A few years later, when Tim was in Las Vegas for the weekend (he drove out there frequently from LA), he bumped into her when she was working as a keno girl. They had a steamy night (actually early dawn) together, and they worked out an "agreement" that he thought would allow him to win more money more frequently. The result of this plot was that Rhonda was now deep into her addiction and got fired by her boss with whom she was also sleeping. Then Rhonda was not only deep into addiction, but also deep in debt. She contacted Tim to tell him that she was pregnant and needed cash, which he sent her weekly for a while. He later found out that she had lied and broke contact with her again.

On another occasion when Tim had been in Las Vegas, he met Sammi who worked "independently" late at night and in certain parts of the city. She had led Tim to believe that her father was a successful surgeon and seemed to have the poise to reinforce that claim. He ended up spending much more on her than if he had had a contract rate because he bought her clothes, paid her bills, and then she stole his credit cards to feed her growing addiction. Tim did not recall where or when he had lost his wallet, so he was unaware of Sammi's deceit. He became a victim of identity theft and had many financial problems.

Tim had been at a party in Santa Monica and had been seduced upstairs by Courtney whom he believed to be "Mireya" because that was her alias for the night. When Courtney became pregnant, she was upset because Tim did not even remember his brief nighttime fling with her, which further angered her. She vowed to be nice to him as long as he gave her money, which he did for a while. He demanded a paternity test which showed a match. She then began to ask for high sums of money. When he balked at paying her so much money, she quietly moved, leaving no forwarding address and got an unlisted phone. She did find his car and poured sugar in the gas tank while deflating the tires. But as her final blow to punish Tim for not wanting her, Courtney anonymously sent a copy of the paternity test to Tim's fiancée.

Tim's fiancée whom he loved dearly then told him where to go and kept the engagement ring.

Tim also started dating Ariana whom he had met through work, but she gave him a venereal disease which was automatically reported to the County.

Around this time, Tim's only brother, Marc-Evan, came out of the closet. Although he had not been so close to Marc, this presented as another stressor in Tim's life. For some reason, around this time also, Tim started to become a sexual compulsive, and brief relationships became the norm. That was followed by compulsive attendance at strip-joints, dialing of "900" telephone numbers, purchases of many porno-movies by cable-on-demand, and a lot of simulated sex on the Internet.

Tim spent his thirtieth birthday out drinking beer and began to realize that his life was slipping away. He continued to roll out to Vegas with his buddies, but one by one, they all got married, and Tim felt lonely. He was driving home alone again from Vegas one night, and his right groin started to ache again. 'Oh no, not NSU again for the fourth time', he thought to himself (Non-Specific Urethritis, a low-grade form of male venereal disease).

Over the next few weeks, he began to feel progressively withdrawn, and did not feel happy when the weekends rolled around. He lost interest in sex for a while and was seeing the world in shades of black, white, and grey. His family started to comment on this, and tried to help Tim. Tim started to spend more time in bars drinking beer and continued to go to Vegas until his debt load became burdensome. Then he stayed home and spent more and more time on the Internet. He might be on-line through the wee hours, and he felt so sex-obsessed, that it consumed him and worsened his Depression.

Discussion: This shows how some people who seem to be most likely to succeed in high school and college can lose their tempo if they become too self-indulgent. Also, his family genetics started to overcome him in young adulthood—these are risk factors which can alter a young person's life. Tim has developed a low-grade Depression along with serious compulsive behaviors. This could also be diagnosed later as a mild Major Depression if he does not curb his downward spiral. The Depression will likely become a chronic mild Depression, dysthymia, because it interplays with his progressive compulsive disorders which are chronic and lead to chronic Depression.

Diagnosis: Tim has Dysthymia that he is self-treating with beer (Alcohol Abuse). He has become a sexual compulsive, also. His brother and sister also have various types of Depression and compulsive disorders.

Outcome: if Tim continues to do the same, he will continue to get the same results: he will start to drink more, he will become puffy and bloated, and then more Depressed. He needs to be in treatment: men's group, SLAA (Sex and Love Addicts Anonymous), and possibly Gamblers Anonymous or Debtor's Anonymous. Luvox might be very helpful.

LOUISE

Louise started to become depressed early in high school, and by the end of high school, she felt mildly Depressed. She always felt about the same: somewhat tired, unmotivated, and feeling like she was out of lock-step with the rest of the world. There were no crippling psychiatric symptoms, but she was only operating at about 70% efficiency at work and with friends and family. Whenever she was Depressed, she felt it as tiredness. It was easy for her to tell people that she was "too tired" for activities, but pride prevented her from exposing her inner vulnerabilities by telling them that she was "too Depressed." Besides that, she did not believe that having one symptom of tiredness qualified as [mild] Depression, anyway. Sometimes, she felt so lackadaisical, that she would take a day off around the end of the week* for feeling "too tired." Not to say that Louise had been an angel: she did try treating herself with various street drugs and alcohol for a few youthful years, all of which left her feeling equally Depressed and sometimes, more Depressed.

She finally landed a job in the trades that provided her with health insurance coverage. She lost little time in finding a psychiatrist who diagnosed her with Dysthymia and prescribed her a series of medications, one by one, each of which seemed "pretty good" for several months or a year, but always left her with some undesirable side effects: Zoloft (not enough quality sleep), Paxil (weight gain), Elavil (weight gain), Celexa (queasiness), Trazodone (morning grogginess), Prozac (rash), Vivactil (rash), and Effexor (persistent elevation of blood pressure). A few mood stabilizers, secondary medications, uncommon antidepressants, and side effect medications had also been tried along the way (Buspar, Vistaril). Occasionally, her psychiatrist told her to take a "drug holiday" (a period of a couple-few months without any medication) after which she would slowly begin to feel "too tired" again. Finally, they hit upon the plan to try St. John's Wort (herb), and it worked excellently!

Diagnosis: Dysthymia with multiple intolerances to synthetic medications

Rx: herbal

Outcome: quite good. Dysthymia typically does not require aggressive treatment or the deployment of powerful medications. In fact, a number of synthetic antidepressant medications may be too strong—including even the "mild" ones (such as SSRI's).

---

*(typical of Depressives who "recharge" during the weekend by oversleeping then cruise through Mondays only to spool down by Thursday, calling in sick on Fridays—unlike alcoholics who oftenest call in sick on Monday mornings after a weekend binge and then really perk up again by Friday as the next weekend nears).

MAJOR DEPRESSION

This one diagnosis probably accounts for more psychiatric appointments than any other single diagnosis. This diagnosis is usually made when there are obvious alterations in emotions, mood reactivity, spontaneity, sleep, and pleasure seeking. Activity levels are decreased and commonly characterized by a sense of generalized slowing, withdrawal, social avoidance, irritability, anxiety, lack of motivation, "shiftlessness," tiredness, and lack of interest in life in general. (See Symptoms in Part One)

Major Depression is the official APA name for a Depression of such significance that a psychiatrist should ideally be involved in all cases. Without professional treatment, the outcome of Major Depression will probably be unpredictable: it will likely fester and get worse, at which point it can morph into a worse case of Major Depression. There might even be a suicide gesture. Other likely possibilities are that an untreated, under-treated, or improperly treated Major Depression will result in attempts at self-treatment with alcohol and drugs (see Part Three, Introduction, last paragraph). There may also be secondary anxiety disorders that develop out of untreated Depressions. All of these potential secondary problems can result in side effects of personality alterations such that the untreated Depressive may expose his friends and family to the "full monty" of his emotional incontinence. Anyone with a Major Depression should see a psychiatrist and not rely upon his family doctor for treatment. If a person is unsure if he has a Minor or Major Depression, then this is another good reason to see a psychiatrist.

Major Depression has different degrees of severity: Mild Major Depression, Moderate Major Depression, Chronic Major Depression, Severe Major Depression, and Severe Psychotic Major Depression. Other subtypes of Major Depression are Agitated Depression and Anxious

Depression. Psychotic Depression is so profound that it is accompanied by one or two psychotic symptoms (loss of contact with reality)—as described below. Agitated Depression is a form of Major Depression that occurs with hyperactivity, inability to be still and sleep well, and a sense of raciness without being manic. Anxious Depression is a combination of anxiety and Depression. In its milder form it may appear as a Reactive Depression that has the formal APA name of "Adjustment Disorder with Mixed Anxiety and Depressed Mood." Post-partum Depression may become a full-fledged Major Depression, but I have listed it separately in this book under "Other Depressions." Major Depression may return on a second occasion. There is also a major type of Depression similar to Major Depression that recurs in a cyclical pattern, (and conforms to certain other diagnostic requirements). This is "Recurrent Unipolar Depression," a form of Cycling Depression. Two other forms of Major Depression, "Double Depression" and "Dual Diagnosis Depression," are covered here at the end of this Section on Major Depression.

KIRK: MILD MAJOR DEPRESSION

Kirk has worked in maintenance for the County school system for twelve years. He has taken extra courses at a community-based Technical Institute, and now feels that he deserves a raise. When he is passed over for a raise, he feels angry inside. Then he broods about this all weekend and refuses to work around the house: 'who cares?' he angrily thinks, 'I have all this extra HVAC training and plumbing skills, what was the purpose of all that training?!' He has trouble falling asleep at night and has low self-esteem. He naps or watches TV all weekend and is not interested in sex, thinking to himself that his wife has become too "pudgy." A month later when his wife is gone for the day, Kirk is so angry after drinking too much coffee that he puts his fist through the dry wall and then has to go to urgent care where he is asked "embarrassing" questions and given the phone number of a psychiatrist. Additionally, Kirk has symptoms of low self-esteem, angry mood, brooding, mild sleep problems, decreased interest in his hobbies, and low sex drive.

Discussion: If he does not see the psychiatrist, his acting-out will worsen, he will have more symptoms, and he will pursue the typical "guy" activities of overeating, drinking, and spending huge sums of money on a new truck, jet-skis, big screen TV, and/or a boat. Then he will have a moderate Depression fed by "buyer's remorse."

Diagnosis: He has a mild Major Depression.

Treatment: He was given low-dose Effexor-XR

Outcome: His anger, anxiety, and Depression improved over the next two months. He slept better, became a better husband, and had better concentration at work. His job performance began to reflect his training; he became very agreeable at work and was later given a raise and promotion. He patched the holes in the dry wall and in his wife's heart and was grateful that he had not hit anyone during this outburst. His sexual desire returned but his performance was marginal; however, he was willing to put up with this in exchange for feeling better (when men say this, they are also telling me how Depressed they had felt: that mental well-being outranks sex). His blood pressure remained normal, but he did develop some mild constipation that responded well to Colace.

IDA: MILD MAJOR DEPRESSION

Ida is a middle-aged executive secretary who gradually started to feel slowed down without reason. She began to lose interest in her job, slept too much, and had no appetite. She also lost interest in gardening, knitting, and cooking. Her family told her that she was slowed down. She started crying every night when she watched TV alone. She began to brood about her husband who had been twelve years older and had dropped dead of a heart attack while taking the Gold Line downtown to work two years ago. She missed him, but did not miss the fact that he had been sleeping with his secretary for the year prior to that.

So she asked her family doctor, Dr. P, for a "nerve pill" and he gave her Paxil 10 mg which she took for a month. When she started to feel better after a month, she quit taking it because she was now 'all better'. Within a few days, the Depressive symptoms came back, so she took it again, but it was not quite so effective, so she went back to Dr. P who reluctantly doubled the dose to Paxil 20 mg and told her to see the psychiatrist, Dr. Z. Since Dr. P had not given her any refills, she was forced to go see Dr. Z three weeks later when she was feeling better. Dr. Z assessed her Depression, increased the Paxil, and told her to come back in three weeks, but she did not return because she was feeling better again and quit taking the prescription when all the pills ran out.

Several weeks later, she felt more Depressed and went back to see Dr. Z who gave her Paxil 30mg, but this time it did not help her and—even worse—it now gave her nausea, itchiness, and irritability. So Dr. Z changed her to Prozac 20 mg which seemed to have the same side effects. She had decided to quit taking Prozac after four days. Later that day she talked to her cousin in Ohio who had been taking Prozac 60 mg with much success. She called Dr. Z and he encouraged her to increase Prozac to 40 mg and come back and see him in ten days. She raised the Prozac but felt nothing. On the morning of the fifth day, she started to feel calm and she told him this at her next appointment with him. He told her to continue the Prozac and within a week she was feeling really well. Well enough, in fact, to fly to Ohio for a week to visit family, during which time she forgot to take her Prozac altogether, because she was so pleasantly distracted on the trip. As a result she returned home feeling well and saw no reason to take any more Prozac.

Ten days later, her Depression returned and she resumed the Prozac, but it did not help. She doubled the dose at home on her own, and then felt agitated. She made another appointment to see Dr. Z who raised the dose to 80 mg over the next three appointments. She felt well again, but began to have insomnia, weird dreams, and jitteriness. Eventually Dr. Z lowered the Prozac to 60 mg and added low-dose Trazodone (antidepressant) at bedtime. She slept well but awoke feeling groggy each morning; Dr. Z halved the dose of Trazodone and added L-Tryptophan; then she slept well and awoke eager each morning.

Then she suddenly developed a rash all over her body. The Prozac was stopped and the rash went away. She tried several other medications, but did not like them as well as Prozac, so she went for a consultation with a dermatologist, Dr. D, who discovered that the rash, apparently, had occurred the morning after eating fresh *ceviche* at a Peruvian restaurant. Then she remembered that she had turned "as white as a sheet" after eating the *ceviche* at dinner and had also felt dizzy and queasy. So he diagnosed a possible toxic seafood reaction and gave her permission to resume the Prozac at 5 mg a day and slowly increase to 20 mg at which time she felt better and then increased the Prozac slowly back up to 60 mg a day with bedtime trazodone. She tolerated all this and felt better.

Discussion: this is a good real-life example of what happens when patients play with their medicines, tinkering with the doses, forgetting to take medicine, and so on. She had originally been stable on Paxil, but by playing around with it, she developed a certain "resistance" to its desirable effects. This also happened with Prozac to a certain degree. Antidepressants that are effective can lift a Depression. If a Depression responds well to an antidepressant for a period of months or years, then, the antidepressant effect might last as long as a month after the medication is stopped, depending upon the Depression and the medication. In Ida's case, the effect did not last so long, because the Depression had not been totally suppressed for a long time, but this case does show that the effects of the medication can outlast the medication itself. If a person does well on an antidepressant for several months then quits it, the drug will pass out of the body within a couple days (a few days for Prozac). However, the medication effects on brain chemistry last longer. A large number of my patients have taken such a medication for such a period of time and then pronounce themselves "cured," whereupon they stop the medication and continue to feel fine for weeks, at which point they convinced themselves that they never had been Depressed and imagine that all the symptoms were "just in their heads." A few days or weeks after that, all the drug's effects on the brain will be gone. In a sizable number of these cases, the Depression returns, as does the rueful patient, to my office. They seem mystified, "I did so well without it for weeks, I don't know what happened." What happened was that the Depression was still present, just suppressed temporarily. It is inadvisable for patients to treat themselves in this way.

As far as rashes, the most serious antidepressant drug rashes occur very early in treatment—within days or a couple weeks. Rashes can occur later in treatment after any dosage increases, especially if the medication has been increased to very high doses. Prozac is often associated with rashes under such circumstances or at the beginning of treatment. However, rashes appearing much later in treatment may not be primarily due to antidepressants, and other causes for the rash should be sought. (Mood stabilizers such as Lamictal and certain other drugs are exceptions and might cause serious rashes in later phases of treatment.)

Diagnosis: (1) mild Major Depression; (2) rash probably related to "seafood allergy" (possibly ciguatera toxin?); (3) diagnosis of "medical noncompliance" when patients take their pills erratically or as they feel the "need" (whenever that might be)—yes this is a real but minor diagnosis and has its own code, V15.81.

Rx: continue bedtime Trazodone without L-Tryptophan—due to her recent rash, she would not be a good candidate for continuing L-Tryptophan with Trazodone and Prozac.

Outcome: good for now; better if she starts following medical advice; although Prozac is well-known for causing a rash, it does not seem to be implicated in this case. (Note: many patients who do self-adjust their medications in this way do not become resistant to the beneficial effects in such a short time period, but this is still no reason to play with the dosages.)

ARIANA: MODERATE MAJOR DEPRESSION

Ariana's parents had always encouraged her to strive for success. While in high school, she became intrigued with the dazzle of the entertainment industry and its "celebrity" status. After high school and college, she moved to Los Angeles where she continued her education by taking many relevant evening courses in The University for several years and started to work her way up in the entertainment industry.

She has scratched and skirmished her way up to a stressful and demanding job in one of the studios in L.A. She likens herself to an electronic gadget in the sense that she is always "on." She goes out almost every evening to hobnob with acquaintances from the entertainment world and maybe talk to or dance with a minor celebrity. On the rare evenings when she is home alone, she feels antsy and restless, so she continues to take more evening certificate programs at The University. If she stays at home alone for even one night, then she worries about what she is missing—and what would happen if she aged without climbing further up the ladder of success. She gets up at 5 AM in order to exercise and is usually spitting nails by the time she arrives at her office. To her "lazy" subordinates she spits out "Get busy! You can rest when you're dead! Today you'll do XYZ for me or else you'll all be de-employed!!"

And that is how her long day progresses as she barks orders to her staff, and consumes large amounts of sinfully dark coffee, while fawning over her superiors and catering to their every whim.

One of her superiors notices her "compelling" management style and compliments her. Her immediate response is, "Even though I seem so in-control, sometimes I feel a little distracted." He suggests that she probably has ADHD (Attention Deficit Hyperactivity Disorder), which is a very popular diagnosis in LA where the members of the entertainment industry routinely receive this diagnosis in the offices of private psychiatrists. This is often an artificial diagnosis that allows the doctor to prescribe amphetamines which function as performance-enhancers and cognitive-enhancers (making people act quickly and talk cleverly, or so people believe).

But Ariana was not wealthy and did not wish to pay a private psychiatrist, so she decided to try one of the psychiatrists on her HMO plan. She went to her first appointment with Dr Z and told him "My boss told me that I need amphetamines for ADHD. I've done a lot of research on line and agree with his findings." After a lengthy evaluation, he made a preliminary diagnosis of mild Agitated Depression (aggravated by environmental stressors). So he started her on low dose Celexa in the daytime and a small amount of bedtime Trazodone as necessary for sleeping. She was really annoyed because she had planned on using amphetamines to drive her to the top of the ladder. She angrily expressed displeasure with this apparently wrong diagnosis, but no amount of posturing and acting-out would produce the desired amphetamine prescription, so she left the office in a huff determined to go on line and report Dr Z's incompetence immediately to the California Medical Board.

Surprisingly, Ariana for some reason started the Celexa and found that she did feel delightfully calm for a few days and then quite buzzy for another couple of weeks. She was pleased and continued this treatment. She continued with doctor Z until her HMO plan changed once again.

Discussion: People working under constant high levels of stress can develop agitated Depression which may be appear with symptoms of poor concentration, irritability, decreased attention span and several other symptoms of Depression. Many adults mistake this for another condition, and many are not even aware of having Depression. Ariana does not have ADHD because this condition starts before age seven; additionally, Ariana has clearly done well in school for thirty years. These constant high levels of stress come from outside sources (environment and jobs) but also from inside us (our self-imposed "need to succeed").

Diagnosis: Agitated Depression due to high stress job and life.

Treatment: Celexa and occasional use of bedtime Trazodone

Outcome: depends upon whether she can control her overpowering need to succeed, but at any rate she continued the Celexa and stopped berating her staff to such a degree that they even invited her out for a birthday luncheon—not because they liked her so much better, but because she was making a noticeable attempt to improve her behaviors.

FLORENCE: SEVERE MAJOR DEPRESSION

Florence was middle-aged. Everything seemed to be going routinely in her life—or at least as far as she knew—when she suddenly started to slow down. The change was neither gradual nor abrupt but was significant enough that she became immediately aware of a decline in her general mental and physical functioning. She did not tell her husband about it, but she did start to confide in her best friend, Millie, who was kept abreast of the decline. Millie observed Florence and confirmed that all this was going down just as Florence described it. After a month, both women became aware that the condition was a Depression that seemed to be worsening.

Florence went to see her family doctor who ran many medical tests that all came back normal, evidence that she had no known medical disorder such as thyroid, cancer, etc. By this time, Florence was experiencing all the following symptoms: losing interest in gardening and cooking, canceling bridge games, crying spontaneously, feeling daytime sadness, napping three hours every afternoon along with oversleeping or under-sleeping at night, daytime sluggishness, and trouble making decisions, as well as having weight loss (155 to 139 pounds). She also felt that she was no longer being a good wife and felt guilty about this, which worsened her self-esteem: she then began to feel worthless and hapless. She wondered if she might have a serious disease such as cancer, despite her family doctor's reassurances after his ordering of further specialized lab tests on her. So, in anticipation of death, she encouraged her husband to go with her to see their lawyer in order to update their Last Will, Living Will, and other such documents. Florence continued to deteriorate: she lost more weight, did not get out of bed usually, and bathed less frequently. Her husband moved into the guest bedroom and did not come home until later at nighttime. Florence felt alone and cursed. She imagined that death was near—or so it seemed to her, as she began reading the Bible and interpreting it literally.

By the fifth time that Florence dragged herself in for her "worried well" doctor appointment, her family doctor had wisely decided to send her to see the psychiatrist, Dr. Ps. She took Millie with her to her first appointment with Dr. Ps., which gave him some information about her personal life: namely, that she had brought her friend instead of her husband. Dr. Ps started her on Effexor-XR of which she required a high dose. She stabilized on this dosage and did well for about a year. During this year, she became more aware of what had been going on in her personal life and these new insights caused her enough concern that Dr. Ps insisted that she also see a therapist. During this time, Florence realized that all had not been going well in her life, and that the foundations for her Depression were probably laid long before she became aware of the Depression. During her first year of treatment, Florence was astonished to learn that they were almost bankrupt due to her husband's sixteen-year habit of betting on the horse races. Also, her daughter-in-law had been having a prolonged affair, with the result that their third grandchild was not biologically her son's; so, her son asked his wife and the third child to go live with her lover. Florence looked back and realized that her son's marriage had been marginal for a long time, but that had gone unperceived by the family. She was also forced to take a look at her own marriage which had long ago become "mechanical" (just going through the motions).

As a result of all this, Florence felt even more Depressed, and Dr. Ps added Remeron at bedtime to help sleep and agitation. The Effexor-XR was increased to a dose above the FDA-recommended daily dosage (such a dosage increase was necessary, and is not uncommon in cases of serious Depression).

Discussion: this case demonstrates that a severe Depression can start out as a severe case—it is not necessarily a neglected case of mild

Depression that festers untreated for too long. This case points out that a severe Depression can have its onset without any particular precipitant. This case also shows that even a severe Depression may respond well to the use of only one antidepressant (likely to be needed in high doses). The only requirement is that the symptoms be major and severe. There is no absolute rule that more than one medication needs to be used to treat a severe Depression; however, it should be pointed out that high-dose Effexor-XR has dual action (on serotonin and norepinephrine), like taking two antidepressants instead of just one. Note also that the Depression had actually been slowly percolating for quite a while—how functional is a marriage where spouses keep serious secrets from each other for many years? The uncovering of this reality in therapy sessions also shows that any Depression can be aggravated by unresolved therapy issues that come to light: do not take this as a recommendation to avoid therapy. On the contrary, all the unresolved therapy issues must be discussed in order to heal and move on with life. As this new information comes to light, it can trigger a Reactive Depression that can push any Depressed patient into a temporary worsening of symptoms requiring addition of more medicine, Remeron, in this case. The fact that her identical twin Phyllis (next case) also had a similar episode near the same age suggests a genetic component. In fact, identical twins have a substantial probability of having the same or similar psychiatric conditions (but not always).

Diagnosis: Severe Major Depression

Treatment: very high dose Effexor-XR (450 mg), Remeron 30 mg in the evening, ongoing psychotherapy and possibly couples counseling (most husbands in cases like this refuse to participate, thereby effectively denying that they have any contribution to the Depression in their wives). It is not unusual for psychiatrists to use extra high doses of Effexor-XR in severe Depression.

Outcome: she will need major medications for a considerable time (years or decades).

PHYLLIS: SEVERE MAJOR DEPRESSION WITH MELANCHOLY

Melancholy *is an additional set of symptoms that can be added onto Major Depression (or onto RUPD, see below). This set of symptoms serves* *to enhance the definition of a Depression and is found mainly in some cases of Severe Major Depression. Phyllis has all the symptoms of Severe Major Depression (like Florence) plus the symptoms of Melancholy, which include: complete loss of pleasure in all activities, very sad mood (worse in the morning), very early awakening in the morning (around 4-5 A.M.), major weight loss, guilty thoughts (but not psychotic guilt), total inactivity (with occasional agitation), and loss of ability to pretend to be happy—not even for an hour.*

Phyllis is the identical twin sister of Florence. Phyllis had similar onset of symptoms, also, although she was a couple years older when she became Depressed and had attributed the episode to her divorce. Similar to her sister, Florence, she had married a man who had "outside interests," but he was not an alcoholic or womanizer. He did, however, like to go to the sports bar with his buddies after work for a drink or two. Occasionally, he was late because he would go to a strip bar after that, usually for a bachelor party or other "special event." He golfed on the weekends and attended as many special sporting events as possible, none of which interested Phyllis. He did call her if he was more than an hour late and made an effort to keep her aware of his location at all times. He wasn't an alcoholic, he didn't gamble or wager away his wages, and he wasn't having an affair; but, he just wasn't there. They were also childless, which was a huge disappointment to him but not to Phyllis.

Phyllis' symptoms developed and progressed in much the same way as those of Florence; however, unlike Florence, Phyllis also developed symptoms of melancholy that worsened her Depression and made it harder to treat. Nonetheless, Phyllis also ended up on the same medications after a couple trials of other medications. After half a year on this combination, she became somewhat more Depressed, and the doctor added very low dose Ritalin which was helpful.

Discussion: Often identical twins will develop the same or similar psychiatric conditions, and will often respond well to the same medications. Phyllis is slightly different because she also has the symptoms of Melancholy. Patients like Phyllis (with Melancholy) are usually so unresponsive that they cannot recite the melancholic symptoms—this information usually has to come from friends and family. Since Phyllis started treatment on her own and came alone to each appointment, her psychiatrist had to infer some of her symptoms and this may be one reason that she had started with a couple different medications before landing on the ideal treatment. She needed a third medication, probably since **Severe Major Depression with Melancholy** is the deepest form of Major Depression, except for Psychotic Depression. In looking back over her story, Phyllis had withdrawn from her husband a long time ago. She could have reached a compromise with him regarding social and sporting events; instead, she merely chose to withdraw completely thereby absenting herself from the marriage, in effect.

Diagnosis: Severe Major Depression with Melancholy (in the past, this was typically a Depression of older age and received the special name of Involutional Melancholia to distinguish it from simple "melancholy").

Treatment: similar to that of Florence: high-dose Effexor, bedtime Trazodone 200 mg, and low-dose Ritalin; Phyllis declined to see a therapist.

Outcome: fair; she will need aggressive treatment for a long time. Being alone after the divorce may worsen the Depression—as we say, "sometimes something is better than nothing" (although it is also sometimes better to be alone than in a bad relationship).

HILDA: SEVERE MAJOR DEPRESSION WITH PSYCHOSIS

We usually refer to this simply as **"Psychotic Depression"** *since it is by definition a Major Depression that is also severe. This Depression is so serious that it is accompanied by loss of contact with reality. This usually means that the person has delusions, illusions, or hallucinations. Delusions are fixed false beliefs that cannot be changed by logical reasoning. (Once the patient gets the delusion in his head, it cannot be removed by anything on earth— but it can be suppressed by antipsychotic medications.) An illusion is a real stimulus but the psychotic patient misinterprets its meaning. Hallucinations occur when a person imagines things that do not exist: like purple elephants in the bedroom at night.* Psychotic symptoms are explained basically under the "Thoughts" Topic in the "Symptoms" Section in Part One. *In Psychotic Depression, delusions are common, illusions do occur, but hallucinations are rare. In Psychotic Depression, the psychotic symptoms usually retreat with the use of anti-psychotic medication and may go away* *for good (unlike in schizophrenia or Psychotic Depression after a stroke, where psychotic symptoms are usually permanent)* .

Hilda's husband, Fernando, has colon cancer. When she learns of his diagnosis and its significance, she becomes very anxious and then becomes agitated. She has trouble sleeping at night, and within a few weeks, she is up all night pacing and praying. She goes to mass every morning and twice on Saturdays. Their HMO tries to cancel her husband's insurance policy. Their son, Abel, is a lawyer and intercedes on their behalf to have the insurance reinstated. Nonetheless, it was a harrowing experience and their insurance was actually voided for one month when Fernando received $19,000 of treatment. Hilda and Fernando receive the bill for this and are forced to pay up, after which the bill can be arbitrated. Hilda is now beside herself with worry and anguish.

Years ago, she had worked full-time and then cut down to part-time. She had later quit working because she was tired of dealing with her boss and the long commute. Now she begins to brood about the fact that she could have kept working for five more years back then with the result that now they would have had an extra $20,000. She begins to blame herself. She is not eating, she is losing weight, and she feels very guilty for their circumstances. She also imagines remembering that Fernando had extra job stress after she had quit her job. He had been so stressed that he started to have heartburn a couple years ago. She is sure that she caused extra stress on her husband's digestion, and that is the cause of the colon cancer. She broods about this constantly, but does not express most of her thoughts, just a few of her conclusions, which seem like disconnected statements to her family who are unaware of the complete libretto of her illogical thought processes. She is often up all night, pacing to and fro. She is restless without knowing why. No amount of reassurance by nurses, doctors, or family will convince her otherwise. She is sure that this whole situation is her divine punishment for quitting her job. And, then she develops heartburn herself, which she assumes is early cancer, another divine punishment meted out to her.

She feels that she must show her God that she is appropriately penitent so she brings broken glass to the cathedral, strews it in the main aisle, and then proceeds to crawl on her hands and knees through the glass all the way up to the altar. She arrives at the altar bleeding, prostrates herself before the altar, and starts to sob and shriek in Latin. Then she lies there muttering Latin phrases. This creates such a stir that the priest calls Abel to come pick her up.

By this time, she has lost weight and sleep, is severely withdrawn, and believes that they are bankrupt and that she is responsible for everything bad. She retreats into her own shut-in world. She asks her husband to forgive her, has irreconcilable guilt, and fears that she will spend eternity with "the Fallen Angel." She hires a neighbor boy to make a little plywood hut in the backyard so that she and Fernando can rent out both the main house and the little guest house in order to make money ($19,000 to be exact). She also believes that she has caused Fernando's cancer. She would like to kill herself, but she is a *creyente* ("believer," devout catholic) and cannot do that—she wonders if she can ever be forgiven for her terrible sins and still go to Heaven. She feels little hope of that. She stops eating, loses weight, and then has heartburn herself, which she assumes is cancer, like Fernando's—her divine punishment. Soon thereafter, she becomes almost non-reactive to her environment and talks very little. She is awake all night staring out the window as if watching for something in the street.

Discussion: Hilda is so severely Depressed that she has psychotic symptoms, namely delusions, which are fixed false beliefs that cannot be changed by logic. These are Depressive symptoms carried forward to their n^{th} degree. Instead of being worried about money, Hilda claims that she is bankrupt and proceeds to behave in exactly that way—she may even abandon her home to go "live under the bridge" because she believes the bankers and sheriff are coming to repossess the house (which she and her husband had paid off three years ago). The police will bring her home from the bridge where they saw her pacing in circles, muttering to herself, and trying to convert the homeless to her religion. She may claim that heartburn is an incurable stomach cancer that must be burnt out of her in which case she may swallow a quart of Listerine or—even worse—bleach. Or she may believe that heartburn is caused by the Devil and therefore must be burnt out of her. She may kill the neighbor's black cat, labeling it as *una cosa del diablo* (a thing of the Devil).

Many years ago, this disease was considered to be a Psychotic Depression that complicated Involutional Melancholia and was well known to respond to moderate doses of major anti-depressants plus low-dose anti-psychotic medications. It is now classified as a Severe Psychotic Major Depression and still responds to the exact same treatment.

Diagnosis: Severe Psychotic Major Depression (the proper APA name for this diagnosis is now "Severe Major Depression with Mood-Congruent Psychotic Features")

Rx: Symbyax (if available on her prescription plan) or generic Triavil (same as Etrafon) or Risperdal plus Trazodone.

Outcome: Fair; the medication will slowly help her symptoms, but she may remain unstable for years, depending upon the outcome of Fernando's colon cancer. She may never recover totally. If Fernando dies from the cancer, she will likely develop an additional Grief Depression and become so psychotically Depressed that she needs psychiatric hospitalization. She will also be at risk for psychosis and Depression if she develops dementia (Alzheimer's Dementia, for example).

DOLORES: CHRONIC DEPRESSION (CHRONIC MAJOR DEPRESSION)

Dolores has been very Depressed for many years. This Depression has interfered with her life in so many ways. She sees her psychiatrist every two months. She has never told him that she also has cocktails in the evening. She feels that alcohol makes her more sociable, although her husband is her only significant social contact. They both have one or two cocktails together in the evening. She has tried many antidepressant medications, secondary medications, and mood stabilizers, and not one of them has helped her very much, for which reason she is now taking three of them. This combination gives her about 40-60% relief, the percentage varying from day to day. She is one of the Depressives who will not get a lot better or a lot worse: she shows "stable instability."

Discussion: There are patients who have tried many medications, but do not respond fully to any medications. These patients are usually given a series of medications and rational combinations of medications that begin to look like doctoring by "trial-and-error." At some point, they often have a modest response and report feeling about 50% better on that particular (and often unorthodox) combination, at which time the dosages are fine-tuned and become the preferred treatment. As a result, patients like Dolores often end up taking a strange concoction of medications which are satisfactory but not great. However, some patients do not respond well to any of the usual—or unusual—antidepressants. These are cases where the patients measure their progress in how much less ill they feel rather than in how much better they feel. Doctors are often willing to go on trying new combinations, but patients become weary of the process and often settle for a 40-60% improvement. This is not a failure on the parts of the patients or the doctor or the drug companies—the best treatment has perhaps not yet been invented (or is simply not available in the USA).

Additionally, alcohol can cause Depression or aggravate Depression. Dolores most probably knows that drinking is a problem, since she has never mentioned it to her psychiatrist over the last fifteen years. Alcohol can have effects on memory and mood and is not recommended for Depressed patients. Patients like Dolores will usually say that drinking is their one main pleasure in life and they refuse to give up their cocktails. Alcohol may not be the primary cause of Dolores' Depression, but she should make an effort to give it up for three months (or switch to dilute wine coolers or "near beer"). As far as likelihoods, the alcohol is likelier to worsen Depression than to improve it. The only way to know the extent of the alcohol's involvement is to stop drinking and observe Dolores' moods and behavior for the following three months.

Compulsive people drink compulsively. If a person cannot quit drinking, then there is some underlying compulsive problem. Asking drinkers to quit drinking is also informative. It is a gauge of their self-control (to be able to quit) as well as an indicator of how serious they think the Depression is. If they are willing to do anything medically reasonable to get over the Depression, then that is an important step—and an indicator of how bad the Depression feels. If they are not willing to follow any medical directions, then that lack of cooperation suggests that they have a compulsive "drinking problem," in which case they need to quit drinking—but these types of patients rarely will. If they are already of retirement age, the doctor may grudgingly agree to provide safe and non-aggressive medical treatment upon the promise that they will "try to" cut down on the alcohol. Younger adults should quit altogether as their drinking puts them at high risk of becoming full-out alcoholics before retirement age—or if not alcoholics, they will at the very least suffer medical problems due to excess daily alcohol, such as liver stress, overweight, diabetes, and many other less common medical complications (hand contractions, bleeding, malnutrition, anemia, all kinds of nerve damage) as well as injuries from black-outs and falls.

Diagnosis and Treatment: Chronic Depression and Alcohol Abuse. If she quits drinking and is still depressed, then she has Major Depression and needs pills. If she quits drinking and feels much better, then she probably had Alcoholic Depression and may need some treatment—perhaps not pills (exercise is a good starting point). If she quits and feels halfway better, then she may have had mild Major Depression aggravated by drinking but not necessarily caused by the alcohol. One or two types of pills may also be helpful in this third case, although three types will not be necessary.

Outcome: can be variable in these cases, but in typical cases, a patient like Dolores will say that she has cut down on the drinking and may end up feeling 50-60% better. But after a while, the drinking may go back to its usual level and she sinks into feeling 40-60% better. This is a good time to add an extra (mild) medication and preface the addition of the new pill by assuring Dolores that the new pill will reduce her cravings for alcohol and will make her feel better overall: frequently, Dolores will indeed feel 60-70% better. Sometimes this improvement can be attributed to pharmacology; and, sometimes, hoping and believing alone may result in improvement.

GEB: "DOUBLE DEPRESSION" (MAJOR DEPRESSION PLUS DYSTHYMIA)

People with Double Depression have special treatment needs in that they will need to have both types of Depression treated simultaneously. Remember that Dysthymia was originally considered to be Depressive Personality, meaning that it is always present and will not go away, thus must be treated. The Major Depression will also need treatment. Since these people have two types of Depression, they usually need at least two types of treatment. Ideally, the Dysthymia could be treated with weekly talk therapy and the Major Depression could be treated with one antidepressant medication. But, unfortunately, it rarely works out this well because of the expense of weekly therapy sessions. Also, at some point in the therapy, there comes a time when all issues have been ironed out, and the personality style remains. Unfortunately, there is no medication that will cure a personality style—it is permanent. Thus, people like Geb almost invariably end up on medium or high doses of one antidepressant (Effexor, for example), or likelier end up on two (or three) medications. Dysthymia is not a federally recognized disability, but Major Depression is; thus, the combination of both, is also a disability. These cases are harder to treat, but not so difficult as Dual Diagnosis (which is Gilbert's story).

Geb had been depressed for most of his life starting with an emotionally tumultuous childhood from which he had never fully recovered. He had not been badly abused at all, but he was an oversensitive person, so that trivial or minor abuses felt magnified. Sometimes the emotional abuse was mainly in his imagination, but his oversensitivity exaggerated it into a minor crisis* (or a *causa belli*). This became even worse throughout his teenage years. All of this left him poorly prepared for life, and he never acquired the basic abilities to be able to pull himself up by his bootstraps. The underlying Dysthymia (see above) became more clinically relevant when he had "senioritis" in his last semester of college at which time he realized that he had spent a lot of money on a liberal arts degree that would never enable him to earn more than a meager salary. During that time, he began to awaken early every morning. He had no control over this awakening, so his only remedy was to go to bed around 8 PM. He awoke every morning plagued by demons from his past, constantly replaying his lifetime's mistakes and imagined injustices done him, which were too numerous to count and a source of constant guilt. These morning Depressive symptoms slowly improved throughout the day until he felt better each evening.

After visiting his family doctor repeatedly because of somatizing symptoms (see Vocabulary at end of book), Geb eventually agreed to see a psychiatrist. He had tried most antidepressants and finally ended up on Ludiomil which seemed to be the best. He continued Ludiomil for years until he started to have episodes of Depression that seemed to resist Ludiomil. The dosage was increased, but eventually Prozac was added to the Ludiomil after which he felt much better and was once again stabilized. He continued like this for several years until it seemed that the Prozac was unnecessary, so it was stopped. He continued on

Ludiomil alone for another couple years and then tried to quit it too, but he felt the dysthymia overwhelming him again. Ludiomil was restarted. After a few more years of taking only Ludiomil, he felt Depressed again and the Prozac was added back with the Ludiomil. Geb felt very good again for several more years until the Prozac seemed to lose its effect and it was replaced with Lexapro. Geb also did well with the combination of Ludiomil and Lexapro.

Diagnosis: Dysthymia in childhood often results in further psychiatric impairments in teenage and adult years. Geb has both Dysthymia and Mild Major Depression; this combination is called "Double Depression." His dysthymia is permanent; his Major Depression came and went and then came back again. The Ludiomil is for the dysthymia. The Prozac/Lexapro is for treating the three episodes of Major Depression. Treatment of Double Depression may require at least two medications or two types of treatment.

Treatment: Geb's psychiatrist continued to prescribe Lexapro with Ludiomil.

Outcome: Geb managed to go back to school to get another degree. He joined Alanon where he found a new understanding family. Geb generally felt good.

---

*even though he was aware of these faux-feelings, he hung onto them obsessively, as if they were minor resentments—this clinging onto faux-feelings and not being able to let go, became his "identified symptoms" (and there was no major emotional abuse), which he freely admitted in therapy, but still was powerless to control.

GILBERT: "DUAL DIAGNOSIS DEPRESSION" (MAJOR DEPRESSION PLUS ALCOHOLISM)

Dual Diagnosis is a special name that is applied to patients who have Major Depression plus Alcoholism (or Major Depression plus Drug Addiction). This is not a formal APA diagnosis, but is routinely used by almost every mental health professional, partly because this diagnosis provides access to extra governmental entitlements and payments—more so than just the single diagnosis of Major Depression (diagnoses such as alcoholism or drug addiction by themselves do not routinely provide access to federal entitlement programs). A person who has this diagnosis has two major illnesses, and recovery from the combination is more than just twice as difficult. Recovery may take three or four times the amount of effort, time, and medical attention. Recovery is complicated by the fact that both diagnoses must be treated simultaneously. If not, then an active untreated Depression can sabotage treatment plans by enticing the addict-alcoholic to start drugging-drinking again in his attempt to self-treat the Depression. If the drug addiction-alcoholism remains active and untreated, then it can cause a Secondary Depression that defeats the antidepressant medication. Dual Diagnosis is also associated with a much higher number of deaths (has more than twice the mortality rate). Death can occur from suicidal Depression or from drug overdose (or alcohol poisoning).

Gilbert had started drinking when he was a "tween" (pre-teenager), which was also about the time that he first started to feel depressed, although in hindsight, he concluded that he might have been "born Depressed." But he was not aware of the depression in those years.

Gilbert joined AA in his mid-twenties and had attained continuous sobriety by age thirty. Gilbert and his sponsor had very fundamentalist beliefs about the practice of sobriety. Thus, Gilbert strongly believed the received AA wisdom that all mood and mind-altering prescription drugs are taboo. Gilbert vowed that he would not take such drugs even on prescription.

After achieving long-term sobriety, Gilbert came to realize that he had been depressed, and also Depressed, for a very long time. He had apprehensively tried two antidepressants for a week each, but he found them ineffectual; they also caused side effects during the first week, which is perfectly normal (these side effects usually start to fade during the second week of treatment). Nonetheless, one week of side effects queered the deal for him, and he refused to take them any longer. He had suspected before trying the antidepressants, that he would not like the effect, and the first-week side effects "proved" him right—at least, in his mind. He also feared that antidepressants would "void" his sobriety. And thirdly, he was also concerned that the antidepressants interfered with the natural state of his brain.

Two of his brothers had committed suicide: one had been a sober drug-addict and the other had been an alcohol abuser. His father had joined AA in middle age and had died a sober death. He had three remaining siblings who had no serious disorders.

Gilbert's wife was frustrated because his mood went up and down: he would be sad then normal then sad then normal, not necessarily in relation to any known factors or stress. Their childless marriage became more of a trial, and Gilbert decided that the world would be better off without him. One day when his wife was at work, he went out and hung himself in the barn.

Discussion: Depression has suicide as a possible outcome, regardless of any other medical, surgical, or psychiatric conditions. And especially, *untreated* Depression can result in suicide. Thus, Gilbert's suicide is not a surprise, but it might have been preventable if he were willing to try an antidepressant for at least three weeks. It is possible that he could have found a serviceable and effective antidepressant.

The AA program was conceived in the 1930's when all psychiatric medications were very addicting, toxic, and potentially dangerous; therefore, AA traditionalists strongly condemn the use of any mind-and-mood-altering drugs, but this is only their unofficial opinion. Despite the historical fact that 1930's psychiatric drugs were addicting, there was/is no official or written policy statement in AA regarding any of those medications, and there is probably a reason for that: one of the founders of AA was a medical doctor. If AA had been conceived eighty or ninety years later, when medications are safer, non-addicting, and relatively non-toxic, then the unofficial stance on these drugs might be different. Traditionalists in AA harshly denounce the use of psychiatric drugs, and this approach is passed down verbally as received "wisdom."

However, nowadays, millions of people can stay clean and sober while taking appropriate doses of appropriate medications prescribed for a legitimate medical purpose. However, such "appropriate" medications should not be addicting drugs or drugs that are cross-tolerant with alcohol—in other words, the drugs should not represent a form of "powdered alcohol." I would consider most non-addicting medications to be safe in recovery and all addicting psychiatric drugs to be risky/taboo. Risky psychiatric drugs include Ritalin, amphetamines, "diet pills," minor tranquilizers, and sleeping pills (Ambien, Restoril, Lunesta, Ativan, Xanax, Valium, Klonopin, and so on). Some addicting drugs have separate uses in neurology, such as Valium, Klonopin, Fiorinal,

Soma, Midrin, and Xyrem; there are usually other non-addicting medications that can be used instead of such drugs. And certainly, the daily use of potent narcotics (for chronic pain) can rarely support the level of serenity needed for high quality sobriety in recovery; examples of such drugs are: Dilaudid, Percodan, Oxycontin, Morphine, and others. There are effective non-addicting non-narcotic treatments for chronic pain. Addicting drugs are all designated with a "C" such as C-II, C-III, C-IV. (see scheduled drugs in Vocabulary)

AA traditionalists, for example, believe that a person (like Marc) who is no longer taking street drugs or drinking alcohol is not genuinely sober, even if he is taking non-addicting psychiatric medication (Effexor). In a sense, the traditionalists are correct: Marc is not in his "natural" frame of mind. If Marc abstained from all psychiatric medications, then he might start to come into focus, but it could take years. If Marc were independently wealthy, he could take all the time that he needs; however, in our frenetic modern society, Marc's not working might mean starving. This is one theoretical basis for putting alcoholics and drug addicts on permanent disability—the only problem is that these patients are not really interested in going back to work—ever; additionally, these patients get bored and end up taking antidepressants anyway while on disability, thereby negating the original goal of giving them a year or two to allow them to find "natural" sobriety.

Diagnosis: Gilbert started early in childhood with a form of Depression (perhaps Dysthymia); apparently, this Depression (Dysthymia) began before or along with the alcoholism, so it is probably a separate diagnosis. He probably drank because he was an alcoholic, we know this from his family genetics; whether he was also using alcohol as a self-treatment for the Depression is not known. Alcoholics drink alcohol because that is what they do—that is their response to any event or issue. They drink because they are happy, they drink when they are sad, and they drink most of the rest of the time, too. Their drinking may or may not have anything to do with Depression. So, now we know that Gilbert by age twenty had both Alcoholism and a form of Depression (probably Dysthymia).

Whether or not Gilbert also acquired a Secondary Depression from primary Alcoholism (Alcoholic Depression) is moot, but most likely he did; the fact that he committed suicide practically demands the existence of a Major Depression: suicide is a severe symptom of Depression, thus it must be associated with a severe Major Depression. Certainly, Gilbert had at least two separate diagnoses: (1) Alcoholism plus (2) Severe Major Depression. If he also had Dysthymia (since childhood) and Alcoholic Depression*, then he theoretically had four different Depressive processes haunting him at all times—remember that alcoholism can be a Depression-Equivalent Disease. Based on his family genetics history, his Major Depression might even have been from a Cycling Depression, such as Bipolar Depression (two/three suicides strongly suggest Bipolar Depression in the family).

Gilbert has many risk factors for Depression and suicide: the risk of suicide in such a case is extremely high. Technically, Gilbert may have had both "Dual Diagnosis" and "Double Depression."

Treatment: he could be listed as a "treatment failure" and perhaps through no fault of his own or of his psychiatrist, who, after all, cannot come over to Gilbert's house every day and force Gilbert to take pills. The old saying informs us that we can lead a horse to water but cannot make it drink. If a person has predetermined that there is a likelihood that no antidepressant will help him, then it probably won't.

Outcome: Gilbert's death might have been prevented if he had been willing to engage in a longer trial of a safe antidepressant, or if his psychiatrist had started him on a mood stabilizer. If Gilbert had been Bipolar, look for a medication response not unlike that of Chet. In general, however, these types of cases have a very high rate of premature death, with very high risk of suicide. If the reader has Dual Diagnosis, he should be certain to avoid all Scheduled drugs: these are denoted by a "C" (CII , CIII, CIV) as opposed to Rx; examples of Rx drugs are non-addicting drugs such as antibiotics, blood pressure pills, diabetes pills, and so on.

---

* one diagnosis of alcoholism does not automatically mean that the same person has a separate diagnosis of Alcoholic Depression—a number of alcoholics may never get Depressed—thus I count these as two separate diagnoses.

CYCLING DEPRESSIONS

(BIPOLAR DEPRESSION, MANIC DEPRESSION, CYCLOTHYMIA, AND RECURRENT UNIPOLAR DEPRESSION)

Introduction: Cycling Depressions (Cycling Mood Disorders) are a family of Depressions that are characterized by having long episodes of Depression that are interrupted by episodes of moods that are not Depressed (non-Depressed episodes) according to this formula:

- the <u>episodes of Depression</u> last for weeks-months-years, usually for many months; during these episodes, the severity of the Depression might be mild, moderate, severe/suicidal, or severely psychotic;
- the <u>episodes of non-Depression</u> last for weeks-months, usually for a few weeks (the non-Depression must last at least four days to qualify as an episode); during the episodes of non-Depression, a person may have baseline mood, or his mood may be joyous, ecstatic, or manic;

The cycling Depressions have an expanded list of terms for describing the mood cycles. The first new term is **Dysphoria**, a miserable feeling, where everything seems out of kilter. Dysphoria is supposed to be the "opposite" of euphoria (which is unconditional happiness). The dysphoric patient sees everything in the world as irritating, gray, and bothersome, no matter what the reality may be. A dysphoric patient may be told that he has inherited a lot of money, and he may respond by being grousy and pessimistic, "Oh, fine, I won't get any of that money anyway after all the government taxes…" The next level of Depression in Cycling Depressions is **Dysthymia** which we already know as a separate Depression Diagnosis. If the dysthymic patient is told that he received an inheritance, he will likely respond by saying, "Oh, I don't care how much money it is: if only it could make me feel happier…" The moderately severe form of Depression is **Major Depression** (as discussed above), and the most severe form of "low mood" is sometimes called **Melancholy** (Melancholia). The melancholic patient might say of his inheritance, "oh now I have something else to feel guilty about… the money won't make any difference because I'll never get out of debt" (even though he has no debt load at that moment). The worst form of Depression in these cases is suicide attempts or completed suicide, which occur frequently in Cycling Depressions.

There is a modern trend in America to over-diagnose Cycling Mood Disorders—this is a common theme of popular daytime TV. Terms such as "Bipolar" are flung about carelessly on talk shows, reality TV, and so on, to the point that the diagnosis is virtually meaningless, since a large fraction of the American population now seems to suffer from some sort of "Bipolar." Pop culture notwithstanding, the proper use of this term needs to be clarified. If a person has little temper tantrums and reacts happily to good news in the morning and reacts angrily to bad news in the afternoon, this is not a Cycling Depression, but rather a series of reactions that do not even add up to a reactive Depression. Neurotic young women and angry men all think that they have Bipolar Depression. This is not true. In most cases, these people have immature personalities and/or drug and alcohol problems. These behaviors do not Bipolar make. Patients who have real Cycling Depressions have very serious disorders that sometimes end in suicide.

The episodes of non-Depression are even more complicated than the episodes of Depression. The weakest level of non-Depression in Depressives is just the baseline mood for that person. In normal people, this baseline is usually called euthymia, but most Depressives are not lucky enough even to have euthymia as their baseline—the typical Depressive's baseline is like a "flat" or blasé mood. **Euthymia** is the "opposite" of Dysthymia. Euthymia, therefore, is a state in which the person feels uniformly satisfied with his life, even somewhat optimistic.

This is the state inhabited by most normal people (non-psychiatric patients). Euthymic patients inheriting money will say "Oh, good, now I can pay down my mortgage and set up a college fund for my son."

One step above euthymia is euphoria, which is the "opposite" of dysphoria (already described above). **Euphoria** is a sense of constant unconditional joyfulness, no matter what the reality is. Euphoric patients inheriting money are just immensely thrilled that anybody would leave them money. They feel delighted and may make plans to travel and buy a time share at the beach. Another step above euphoria is **hypomania**. Hypomanic patients are very active, busy talking and making plans, not sleeping a lot, and taking on all sorts of extra duties, responsibilities, or part-time jobs. They may spend a lot of time "partying" and sleeping around indiscriminately. They become "party animals" living in the "fast lane." If they receive an inheritance, they may buy a sports car (on credit), buy a beach home (on credit), run out to Las Vegas, and gamble away a lot of money on poker and "night life." There will also be modest spending sprees characterized by "maxing out" all lines of credit. But at no time, is their behavior "extreme"— although their spending habits may resemble those of some "normal" modern Americans, the diagnosis of excessive spending should rest on abnormally excessive for that particular patient's baseline spending habits. Worse than hypomania is **mania** in which patients are extremely over-activated to the point of being half-psychotic. They talk so much that they are hoarse; their thoughts are flying so fast, that speech cannot keep up and their interpersonal communications sound like linguistic Morse code or just jabber. They have so many plans, that they can initiate none of them. They go for days seldom sleeping, and may have minor psychotic symptoms such as delusions and illusions (see Psychosis topic in Symptoms Section in Part One). They imagine themselves to be important and at the head of vast enterprises. If they are told that they have inherited money, they would have no idea what that really meant but would be ecstatic, nonetheless; they would be too disorganized to fill out all the paperwork to enable themselves to access the money. They would, however, be involved in all sorts of problems, like manically driving on sidewalks to bypass traffic congestion, and committing many other unacceptable social behaviors that would result in their meeting many new people, some of them wearing blue uniforms (amphetamine addicts may act manic, but they do not have real clinical mania—as soon as the drugs wear off, the drug addict collapses into fatigue). The manic's inheritance would eventually be used to pay for psychiatric hospitalizations and legal fees. If the manics could access the inheritance beforehand (before the manic phase), it would be squandered in very irrational ways on bizarre "projects" during the mania. Manics may (try to) talk themselves onto a first-class seat to Paris without even having a passport, money, or airline ticket. And then they may decide they do not wish to go to Paris and try to open the airplane hatch in mid-flight above the ocean. Manics may go running naked down the street screaming ecstatically in the wee hours. Mania is the "opposite" of melancholy. Manics feel so good that they do not ever wish to kill themselves, but all their antics may result in self-injury due to their poor self-care and total lack of common sense. Unexpectedly, they may die as a direct result of their own actions, which is technically suicide ("suicide" means "self-killing" in Latin.) They may also die as an indirect effect of their actions or of actions that they had previously initiated. (Mania has been further subdivided into various degrees of **ecstasy, elation,** and **exaltation**, but that is beyond the scope of this book.)

In **Recurrent Unipolar Depression**, RUPD, a person has repeated episodes of Major Depression alternating with just his baseline blasé mood—he has no "high" moods (see below). **Cyclothymia** is a rather mild form of Bipolar Depression characterized by episodes of dysthymia and euphoria.

So, the four main Cycling Depressions are: Bipolar Depression, Manic Depression, Cyclothymia, and Recurrent Unipolar Depression. Rapid-Cycling Bipolar and Bipolar-NOS are two more types not covered here. Furthermore, there is a seventh and special case, Borderline Personality Disorder, which has a large number of psychiatric symptoms as well as repeating episodes of Dysphoria and episodes of Depression. So now we can classify mood alterations of Cycling Depressions in this way:

- Cyclothymia = dysthymia ⇆ euphoria
- Recurrent Unipolar Depression = Depression ⇆ baseline personality
- Manic Depression = Mania ⇆ Depression
- Bipolar Depression = Hypomania ⇆ Depression

- Borderline Personality = Dysphoria ⇆ baseline ⇆ mild Bipolar

Bipolar refers to the fact that the moods swing up and down between two "poles", Depression and mania. Unipolar refers to the fact that there is only one pole, the Depressed pole. Cyclothymia may also appear as dysthymia plus mild hypomania. These are only sketchy details on Cycling Depressions—for more details, see my other books *Everyone's Everyday Guide to Practical Psychiatry* and *Defeating Depression*.

Many of these cycling patients also have an ample family history of Cycling Mood Disorders. Such a diagnosis is further supported by having family members with Depression-Equivalent Disorders (ADHD and compulsive disorders, notably alcoholism). The cycling may not resemble the cycling of the seasons of the year, but rather it is "irregularly regular," occurring in certain patterns that are characteristic for that patient. An episode of Depression or of non-Depression may be set off by some environmental disruption or stress, although in many cases, these patients cycle on some unknown basis.

The treatment of Cycling Depression is difficult because the Depression is usually in flux, cycling into a different phase of Depression or non-Depression and rarely remains fixed. So, the treatment goal is two-pronged: to dampen the mood cycles and then to defeat the Depression. The cycling nature of these disorders requires using mood stabilizers with or without antidepressants. Cyclothymia is usually treated with antidepressants. RUPD likewise definitely requires vigorous treatment with antidepressants. However, in manic Depressives, antidepressants can trigger an episode of mania (this is not good). The use of antidepressants in Bipolar Depression patients is very complicated—in a number of research studies, antidepressants have been shown to have little positive or negative effect on Bipolar Depression. In some cases, antidepressants can aggravate the non-Depression phase; in other cases, antidepressants might provide modest benefit.

In all cases, staying abreast of the Depression and anticipating its next move is difficult. The most effective treatment is to find one or two medications (antidepressants, mood stabilizers) that work well in that patient and then to fine-tune those medications in a timely manner, depending upon the mood cycle. During extremes in the cycle, a third or fourth medication may be added temporarily to dampen the cycling. If a patient can stay with the same doctor for many years, the doctor may be able to get good control of the cycling, although there will often need to be periodic up or down adjustments of some of the medications. The reader can now see that Cycling Depressions are hard to treat, and there are psychiatrists who specialize only in mood disorders.

111

CYCLING DEPRESSION
BIPOLAR DEPRESSION

Bipolar Depression is characterized by extremes of moodiness ranging from near-suicidal (Depression) to irritable, flat, or joyful upswings. Bipolar Mood Disorder usually first appears in young adulthood and the first episode can be hypomania or Depression. Bipolar that first appears as a Depression can present itself like any of the types of Depression, usually mimicking a Major Depression—yes, that makes it harder to recognize, which is why psychiatrists must always maintain a "high index of suspicion" that a first-time new-onset Depression in a young adult could be a serious Depression. The suspicion can be based on the fact that symptoms that have appeared from nowhere and are not due to any known cause, or the only cause being genetic which is invisible and not routinely screened—yet. If it is genetic, then the only clue might be from family history. This Bipolar Depression may often appear rather quickly and may promptly become a moderate Major Depression. Other possible warning signs that we are in the presence of Bipolar Depression (and not an ordinary Depression) would be age of onset (late teens or early twenties), extensive family history (of Depressions, mania, alcoholism), as well as a personal history of extreme irritability, suicide attempts, and unusual responses to antidepressants (extreme irritability, sudden euphoria, or sullen and persistent Depression when exposed to antidepressants). Patients presenting with their first Bipolar episode as a Depression usually have an unusual response to the first-time use of antidepressants. They may become hypomanic within a matter of days or they may dive deeper into a seemingly prolonged Depression characterized by an internal restlessness—they may feel wound up inside but "nothing is coming out," like a high revving car stuck in "Park": the

Bipolar Depression is weighing them down while the antidepressant is giving them internal stimulation that cannot express itself externally due to the (temporary) weight of the Depression. These "high revvers," however, will sooner or later burst forth into high gear, and this could be a very dramatic event.

Family doctors who are obliging enough to treat an apparent "Minor Depression" can sometimes be surprised when these patients lapse into a hypomanic episode which can sometimes evolve into a psychiatric emergency. Even psychiatrists are sometimes caught off guard by a few of these cases. The best way to diagnose this possibility is by being watchful and collecting a great deal of information on the new patient before prescribing any new medications. The most important information is family history and the story of how the patient (like Chet) came to be Depressed. Being watchful might mean seeing the patient more frequently, perhaps even twice a week early in treatment.

Long-term stability is possible if patients are willing to communicate often and freely with their doctors. One big problem occurs in cases where patients are not good observers of their own behavior. In these cases, they feel that they have nothing to report. These people are problematic because they are prone to relapse unless they are willing to come in and see the doctor frequently—and most of them choose not to do that. They have unstable courses and are re-hospitalized. Other problems may occur whenever patients make certain unwise personal decisions. They may decide that they are tired of taking synthetic chemicals, tired of being ill, tired of seeing psychiatrists, or tired of the stigma of psychiatric illness. They may decide that they should will themselves to be well. They may think that yoga, athletics, magnets, sunlight, travel, geographic relocation, herbs, omega fish oils, or some other method can control them. They might want to spend their junior year abroad and quit all medications, pretending (denying) that they even have a mood disorder. Occasionally, bipolar patients may deliberately quit medications in order to lurch into a hypomanic episode that will give them an energy boost so that they can finish graduate school, run the LA marathon, or work extra hard on a big project at work. They may decide that they like the euphoria of being hypomanic and decide to quit their mood stabilizers. They will eventually become hypomanic but then fall into a serious Depression after that. Then they might become so Depressed that they feel suicidal: suicidal because of the biochemical effects of the Depression on their brains, suicidal because their disorder is hard to stabilize, suicidal because they want to be hypomanic all the time and cannot, suicidal because they are tired of being "mental," or suicidal over other problems in their lives which are tinged dark by the Depression, thereby obscuring their judgment and ability to observe their life-situation objectively. There are several routes that might lead from Bipolar Depression to suicide—not just one.

A few people have money issues: they do not have the money for an office visit. Or they do have the money for an office visit, but think that psychiatrists do not "do" anything therefore do not earn their pay; perhaps the doctor visit is worth $10 to the patient but he balks at paying $35. There may be resentment that psychiatrists make money from other people's unhappiness, or patients may have some other financial issues.

Not uncommonly, patients resent organized psychiatry but like their psychiatrist as a person. There are still other patients who are willful and do not want anyone else telling them how to live or what to do—especially psychiatrists; these patients are suspicious that psychiatrists are somehow controlling their minds or "manipulating" them. We psychiatrists do need to "manipulate" people like this: manipulate them into trying to be well. In the same way that dentists try to "manipulate" people into flossing everyday. These issues are all rooted in a patient's personality style. A patient's course and stability ultimately depend upon overriding and subduing any of these stubborn personality factors that might interfere with recovery. Psychiatrists try to work with people to overcome these issues; if that is not successful, then they are often referred to a therapist or psychologist. If all this fails to remove personality problems that obstruct a patient's recovery, then he should consider finding a psychiatrist—any psychiatrist—whom he feels he can trust (changing doctors rarely changes a patient's personality). If the patient cannot rein in his obstructive personality issues, then they become destructive personality issues: his outcome is not so rosy. Not rosy at all.

In contrast, there are a variety of people with all types of Cycling Depressions who may remain relatively stable on the same dosages of the same medications for years on end; these patients need but little tinkering with their medication(s) over the long-term. One of the main reasons for changing their mood medication(s) might be related to the development of a new medical illness that requires starting new medical medications that conflict with the mood medications. For example, a bipolar patient Rudy has been taking Depakote successfully for years, but then gets Hepatitis-C from a lover; the Depakote should not be used with hepatitis; Rudy will need to take hepatitis treatments, all of which can cause Depression; Rudy might need an antidepressant, but antidepressants can aggravate bipolar patients; Rudy might need to switch to Lamictal, unless there is some reason he cannot take Lamictal, and so on. At this point, Rudy, and his liver doctor and psychiatrist need to make a three-way decision on which medications to use. Most psychiatric and medical medications have alternates—but not always. Or, another problem in taking one stabilizing mood medication for a long time is that the mood medication might be putting undue stress on the organs of the body; this happens with manic Depressives (Hank) who have taken lithium for many years: even though the lithium has served Hank well, eventually the lithium will start to cause him kidney or thyroid problems requiring him to change to Depakote or Tegretol.

Apart from all this, another problem is that Bipolar Disorder is being seriously over-diagnosed nowadays, sometimes to the point that the diagnosis can apply to almost any mood condition or moodiness, tantrums, compulsive behavior, character instability, or personality disorder. Some psychiatrists and psychiatric clinics seem to diagnose 20-40% of all their patients as bipolar nowadays, which seems wildly excessive (as little as three decades ago, the number was under 1%). This diagnosis is applied equally to people with many types of mood disorders, personality disorders, alcoholism, or drug-addiction. It is not uncommon for me to see new patients coming from "St. Elsewhere" where they have been given the diagnosis of bipolar, but are not taking any standard treatments for bipolar. Some of them may be taking only Paxil 20 mg per day or a drug like Valium, neither of which are an acknowledged treatment for Bipolar disorder. Some of them may be taking only Prozac which can make real Bipolar patients manic and rageful. In these cases, the disorder and symptoms need to be scrutinized carefully—and perhaps the diagnosis needs to be re-worked or changed to a more accurate diagnosis.

This modern trend towards over-diagnosing makes doctoring more difficult because the psychiatrist now needs to sort out the true Bipolar patients from all the pop-culture "wanna-be's" who have seen Bipolar discussed and liberally advertised on daytime talk TV. These people have a very "soft" bipolar diagnosis at best. And perhaps the worst problem occurs in prescribing powerful Bipolar medications to people who do not really need them—and as a result do not tolerate them well, which results in the curiosity of "paradoxical over-medication." This curiosity happens in this way: a person with a drug-and-alcohol problem and immature personality is diagnosed as "Bipolar" because of self-reported moodiness (drug withdrawal), lethargy (hangover / "crashing"), and acting-out (drug intoxication), all symptoms caused by street drugs and alcohol. The person is prescribed Depakote that makes him too sleepy, so the doctor adds Prozac to make him alert enough in the presence of Depakote so that he can continue on Depakote, the need for which is highly questionable in the first place, but at any rate, now he is on two medications. But the Prozac does not take effect for a couple hours each morning, so the person is also given a low dose of Wellbutrin to "goose" him in the morning. As a result of taking two antidepressant medications, he has trouble falling asleep, so is given a Valium-like drug (Klonopin) at bedtime which gives him mild withdrawal symptoms the next day that look like moodiness, and so the Depakote is increased, and so on. And he continues secretly to take drugs and alcohol. This person is at risk of liver damage from Depakote and mixed drug reactions, when his ideal treatment might have been simply to join Narcotics Anonymous instead. (The real reasons for current over-diagnosis concern money and are discussed at some length in my first two books.) Some of these patients are quick to blame their disease: "Oh, my bipolar made me do it" (haven't we heard this plea before, as in "Oh the devil made me do it!") If we are talking about the devil making Rhonda steal her mother's diamond and pawn it to buy cocaine and amphetamines, then that's just Rhonda and her addiction, not her bipolar. This is clearly Rhonda's scheme to acquire money and represents a logical act to benefit Rhonda. This is in contradistinction to the insanity of true bipolar patients who do bizarre things that are meaningless or even detrimental to themselves in which the acts do not represent some sort of logically evolving scheme. The cases shown here below are those of people with legitimate Bipolar Depression.

CARRIE-BETH

She had cried a lot as a baby and had been a somewhat anxious child, but was also prone to episodes of "dramatics." She performed excellently in school plays, but she also went through weeks-long periods when she would feel shy and withdrawn. She did not have social poise, often blurting out off-color stories and acting like hyperactive boys. She did not have ADHD—or at least her superior grades did not suggest this. She would feel very tired and sad every year in January and February. In college she felt very dismal in the fall semester, and then very happy in the spring semester. Her grades were usually quite good except when she had brief "fits" of Depression that prevented her from studying. Finally, she had the onset of obvious mood changes in her early twenties.

She would do exceptionally well at work for a few months, then would sink into a deep apathy and lose all the acclaim that she had earned. Sometimes this apathy resulted in her being terminated from jobs. She would sleep ten hours each night and nap a lot on the weekends when she would stay home and watch romantic comedies in the hopes of motivating herself. When she was productive at work, she was exceptionally animated and bright. During these times, she was very active every weekend and awoke early every day to go exercise. She would accomplish many difficult tasks during these productive times which lasted for a few months, each. At these times, she only slept four-five hours per night. She was almost engaged twice during two of these episodes, but in the ensuing down moods, could not maintain a relationship, or the young men expressed concern at her moodiness which they thought went beyond the tolerable boundaries of mere femininity. Despite all these goings-on, she refused her mother's strong suggestions to see a psychiatrist. She did, however, agree to talk to her family doctor who gave her a small Prozac capsule which (unbeknownst to him) she took only on days when she thought she was Depressed.

She persisted in this "Prozac Experiment" during which time she was able to maintain a semblance of mood stability that allowed her to get into a third long-term relationship with someone who, unfortunately, was 'not as good a catch as the two that got away.' Thus she was engaged a third time, while in one of her "great" moods (euphoria). However, a couple weeks before her planned wedding, she became decidedly worse than at any time in the past. She was extremely hyper-excited, and boarded a plane for Buenos Aires where she wanted to have a last fling ('Last Tango in B.A.', she called it) and go on some sort of spree. She overspent on her credit cards and picked up young men around the city. She became so inappropriate there that she was placed in jail overnight and then escorted to the airport by the police and American consul on the next day. After landing at LAX, her family took her to a large well-known hospital with a psychiatric ward where she was given Depakote and Seroquel. She calmed down within a week, and was discharged a day before the wedding. (Her new husband thought about annulling the marriage but stayed with her until the next year when he divorced her.)

Over the next few years, she was well maintained on moderate-dose Depakote alone. If she became agitated, she would add Seroquel at bedtime. If she needed Seroquel for more than a few days, then she would take Topamax at bedtime to prevent weight gain from the Seroquel. If she had Depressive periods, then she would take half of the smallest tablet of Wellbutrin daily for three weeks—all under medical supervision. She maintained close contact with her psychiatrist and actually remained stable for years. Her moods gave the outward appearance of remaining stable while the medications were manipulated in anticipation of mood changes or in response to medical attempts to abort any serious mood swings.

Discussion: this is a rather typical case and highlights the complexity of treating cycling Depressions: there is a constant need to stay abreast of evolving symptoms while trying not to overmedicate patients. And this is a case that works out well because Carrie-Beth works well with her doctor by keeping him abreast of her thoughts and feelings. Her third fiancé might have been only her third choice as well as being someone to whom she hopefully clung while in an antidepressant-confused state punctuated by fluctuating levels of judgment (Prozac should be avoided in such cases because it can induce mild hypomania characterized by judgment lapses).

Diagnosis: Bipolar Depression

Treatment: Rx medications as listed above.

Outcome: this is a classic case of patients who can maintain stability if they can rein in all their other issues. She can remain stable on a mood stabilizer (Depakote 1000 mg), occasional secondary medications (Seroquel 25 mg, Wellbutrin 37½ mg), and side effect pills as needed

(Topamax 25 mg). She may continue like this for decades; medications may be changed out if newer improved medications come to market. She may have very few or no future psychiatric hospitalizations *as long as* she is willing to trust in the feedback from her doctor and family.

CLAIRICE

Clairice grew up in Cleveland and came from a family well known for moodiness. Her own moody father was a successful entrepreneur, as well as being a "functional" alcoholic. She was a good student and enjoyed singing and ballet. She had a sudden dip in her school grades for a six-week period but then her grades came back up again. When she was fourteen years old, she began to experience a strange and calming effect from the seasonal change in the fall months. She felt quiet and thoughtful at this time of year, and liked to stay indoors reading and writing poetry. She also felt strangely content and did a lot of outside reading for most of her classes, staying consistently on the reserve honor roll. During this time, however, she had much less physical energy. She would continue in ballet and girls' soccer, although her performance was lackluster during this time. By springtime, she would be lively again and resume singing but would do less outside reading for her coursework.

In the September when she was fifteen, she had a superficial relationship with Phil the captain of the baseball team but he seemed somewhat insensitive and then broke up with her in October. Clairice had a prolonged "quiet" episode that Fall which lasted until Christmas. And then she came out of it on Christmas Eve. In the spring, she started practicing with two other girls and they formed an amateur singing and performing trio. They performed at a few local venues and high schools and enjoyed some popularity. Phil wooed her back and convinced her to go out with him again, and then he dropped her again for unknown reasons. Clairice went into such a Depression that her parents took her to see a psychiatrist who referred her for talk therapy with a counselor. Her Depression seemed out of proportion to merely being jilted by another teenager in the sense that it took her months to recover emotionally. Despite good grades, popularity, and a new and "better" boyfriend, she decided one day to take twelve aspirin pills for no apparent reason. Even she had no idea why she did this. She did not mention this to anyone until her next doctor's appointment at which time her psychiatrist then set her up with a psychotherapist and started to prescribe her low-dose Lexapro.

Therapy and Lexapro did nothing and she actually became more and more dysphoric until two weeks later when she took a whole bottle of Lexapro along with as many bottles of cough syrup as she could find. This resulted in her hospitalization where the Lexapro dose was doubled then tripled. She became much more dysphoric and then irritable, complaining that she could not sleep and her brain would not "turn off." Her body felt "immobilized" and yet she could not even fall sleep—she imagined that she was awake all night. So, she was given strong bedtime medications that were hardly effective—she felt revved up but knocked out. In the daytime, she watched TV nervously without having a good understanding or recall of the programs, news stories, or movie plots. She talked about suicide in the hospital until one day when she awoke before dawn full of great energy and boundless excitement. From that moment on, she was so gleeful and euphoric that she was literally bouncing off the walls of the hospital. She had to be physically restrained in the "Quiet Room" (with padded walls), the Lexapro was stopped, and she was started on Depakote, a mood stabilizer. After three more weeks she was stabilized and went home with her parents. She felt good for the first time in quite a long time.

Three months later, she became Depressed again, so that a low dose of a mild bedtime antidepressant (Trazodone as needed) was added to the Depakote. She continued with all her activities, earning good grades and singing with her group at more "gigs." Surprisingly, her new boyfriend stuck by her through all of this. Then she had a second episode during which she felt somewhere between euthymic and euphoric. The doses of medications were adjusted and she felt well for a year at which time she had a second Depression for no apparent reason. As a matter of fact, at that time she was accepted into Prestigious University and her singing trio made a demo recording. In the summer after her junior year at college, she became hypomanic: her Depakote was increased and Trazodone was stopped; then she became quite Depressed and Lamictal was added. She came out of the Depression and stabilized.

Her life continued like this for many years, punctuated by mildly cycling mood episodes that appeared (to other people) as mild Depression episodes and mild euphoric episodes that were rendered tolerable and mild only because she was continuously medicated.

Discussion: this is an example of how Bipolar Depression can begin like a Major Depression and how it may have a delayed hypomanic reaction to the introduction of antidepressants. (This also posits one explanation for suicidality in young people treated with SSRI antidepressants—when they start to emerge from Depression is the precise moment at which they are likeliest to attempt suicide.) This is a Bipolar Depression that responds well to the usual treatments but follows the usual up and down cycles which are acceptably dampened by the medications which nonetheless need periodic adjustments. The reader can see that the medications have a dampening effect on her "emotional roller coaster." Depakote can be taxing to the liver: this side effect is a bigger concern in children than in adults. Since Clairice is a teen, her liver function tests and Depakote blood levels may vary; typically teenagers use up a lot of Depakote, unlike children; at any rate, because of her age, blood tests should be checked frequently.

Diagnosis: Bipolar Depression

Treatment: Depakote controls the up's and down's of mood and Lamictal is helpful in preventing Depressions. She also found Light Treatment (photo-therapy) helpful, since her episodes had started in the fall, and seemed to be aggravated by winter. Eventually, phototherapy, Depakote, and Lamictal were her three main treatments; Trazodone was rarely needed except for serious insomnia. She later moved to Florida and rarely had any more need for Light Treatments.

Outcome: she is doing as well as possible. Suicide risk is present, especially since she had already made two minor gestures as a teenager. This establishes that overdosing is her preferred manner of acting out her Depressions. Her family history suggests that she has the genetic underpinnings for Cycling Depression, as well as for possible alcoholism (plus the fact that her second overdose attempt was with cough syrup containing alcohol).

She later had a serious post-partum Depression after her first baby, which was even worse after the second baby. The Light Treatment had never made her hypomanic, but it could have.

Bipolar Depression with Dysphoria in Borderline Syndrome

(Also Called Borderline Personality Disorder)

People are basically born with this disorder. Starting after birth and throughout life, these people go through "relational extremes": they need constant love and yet never get enough and are incapable of reciprocating (giving back love). They fall in love quickly and fall into hate just as quickly. But, falling into despair is just as likely—this occurs frequently in the form of recurrent dysphoria. These patients have extreme emotional instability. Whenever they are introduced into a group of people (such as attending school or working in an office), they can cause great upheavals in group relationships and disruptions in schedules and orderliness. People like Courtney may classify new acquaintances into people who either love or hate her. She may not begin each new relationship assuming that every new acquaintance is a "neutral" starting point or a blank slate of new opportunity for interpersonal bonding. Her main system of dealing with people is to manipulate them (based on her first impressions). Courtney may have periods of intense rage directed outwardly to the whole world. This rage shows up as tantrums in childhood, as severely rebellious and prolonged outbursts in teenage years, and as antisocial acting-out in adulthood. The acting-out episodes in adulthood can be directed toward other people but are just as likely directed inwardly, toward herself, which appear as suicide attempts.

As infants, borderline people cry too much, do not sleep well, and need a lot of attention. As children, they have emotional instability, irritability, and tantrums. As older children, they cannot soothe themselves—they need some other person to give them great amounts of attention and care. In order to get this attention, they may put on an act of being solicitous and ingratiating with adults; if this does not produce unconditional love, then they may have a tantrum in retaliation for not getting the attention they crave. These children seem unruly and disruptive at times and may be diagnosed with ADHD, but ADHD falls far short of the real problem of Borderline Syndrome. Dysphoria appears in late childhood, then "soft" bipolar symptoms appear in the teen years, followed by the full-blown Syndrome. It is usually diagnosed in women, but some men may have some or all its symptoms, too—but in somewhat gender-modified form.

This disorder has been studied mainly in women: all the women with this disorder may have different modes of outward expression and apparent operation, but the central emotional problems that drive them are all about the same. They make minor overdose gestures, have episodes of great moodiness, sometimes feel psychotic very briefly, and have stormy relationships with authority figures and other people—especially with men.

The main treatment is weekly sessions of talk therapy with a (female) therapist who sometimes receives the brunt of an occasional angry outburst. Clients such as Courtney view their therapists as mother figures, authority figures, and friends, none of which is real or accurate. During therapy, Courtney will come to learn which role the therapist plays, and that the therapist is a person equally deserving of the same respect that Courtney angrily demands for herself. This whole process takes many years. These clients like Courtney usually start off loving the therapist, but if the therapist does or says something trivial or innocent that enrages Courtney, then there will be an episode of anger directed outwardly or inwardly. The degree of anger will be completely out of line with the imagined slight. If the anger is directed inward, there will be a small suicide gesture or threats of suicide. A suicide gesture or threat serves a double purpose of letting off steam and punishing the "bad" therapist. The therapist is "punished" because the therapist will have to make herself available for extra sessions and phone calls to soothe Courtney—or the therapist will have to go through the whole process of getting Courtney into a psychiatric hospital for a few days of observation ("suicide watch"). If the anger is directed outward, Courtney might call the therapist's answering machine and leave messages full of anger, resentments, and profanity. Courtney might have a sullen, angry, resentful, or sarcastic confrontation with the therapist—or may deliberately "no show" to the next appointment. Courtney will then wait for the therapist to call inquiring about Courtney's well-being—or at least the therapist is "supposed" to do this (therapists are well aware of the ramifications of calling or not calling, and the Courtney's know this, too). If Courtney is very fragile or in early phases of treatment, then the therapist will probably call. If this is a bad habit of a client who is in long-term therapy, the therapist might not call, as a way of setting boundaries. Or Courtney may take all the anger and direct it outwardly at some unwitting victim instead of at the therapist (called "displaced anger"). At any rate, over years of therapy, the borderline client will (hopefully) come to learn how to have a normalized relationship with the therapist; this experience can then be applied to relationships with regular people in Courtney's life. The main treatment is talk therapy which is needed for years or decades.

The doctor has only two minor roles: pills and hospitalization. Doctor visits are quite brief and concerned mainly with pills. Medication treatment visits may be at regular intervals, but are often on an "as-needed" basis, since there are no drugs that will cure this disorder. Courtney may have a very short psychotic episode ("micro-psychotic" episode) deserving of an anti-psychotic medication; she might also have a mini-manic episode that might need a tiny dose of a mood stabilizer. In all such situations, Courtney should be given only tiny amounts of safe medications, because all prescriptions will be hoarded until such time that they will predictably reappear during a suicide gesture. The main focus of treatment for patient, therapist, and doctor is dealing with each new wave of dysphoria that may be accompanied by renewed threats of self-injury (suicide threats). The doctor's other minor but important role is to hospitalize patients like Courtney when they need a "time-out." This is usually related to escalating dysphoria and renewed threats of self-injury. In these cases, three to four days in a hospital is usually the correct amount of time required to defuse the situation. (If Courtney stays too long in the hospital, she will start to disrupt therapeutic relationships of hospital staff with non-borderline patients and possibly cause other interpersonal relational problems. Once this happens, it is a sign that Courtney is back to her "normal" baseline behavior and ready to go home).

The doctor is not uncommonly a male physician, whom the borderline patient may perceive as her father figure, uncle figure, or authority figure, which also is not realistic. However, this set-up often works out well, because Courtney may perceive her female therapist and male physician as substitute "parents." This may provide Courtney with the opportunity to be "re-parented." Most of these clients have had distorted relations with their parents: often their own mothers are borderlines who despise men, whereas their own fathers are detached, absent, or "hen-pecked."

Well over half of borderline patients report childhood memories of physical or sexual abuse. If they have not experienced these two types of abuse, almost all of them most surely have at least had emotional abuse (growing up with a borderline mother, for example). The source of the sexual abuse might be the fathers, but is just as likely—or likelier—to have been anyone else: uncles, grandfathers, cousins, elder brothers, neighbors, boyfriends, and so on. Toward the end of the twentieth century, there were reports that some of the "retrieved" memories of sexual abuse in these patients might have been exaggerated by the patients or might have been encouraged by certain female therapists (with their own personal untreated sexual abuse issues). Since borderline clients are known for having overactive imaginations, some of the sexual abuse memories might have been "enhanced" experiences of childhood curiosity that could have been within normal limits. Courtney may have had natural curiosity about a boy close to her own age, and may have amplified and distorted this whole encounter—these patients can also be suggestible if a therapist asks too many leading questions. In some cases, their mothers might have told the clients that their fathers gave them baths occasionally, and this could have been subconsciously "upgraded" into the possibility of forgotten episodes of fondling. Thus far, sexual abuse has not been proven to cause Borderline Syndrome.

Regardless of cause, Borderline Syndrome involves serious emotional instability and distortions of interpersonal relationships along with some skewed reality interpretation.

Borderline Depression refers to the many Depressive aspects of Borderline Personality. The first aspect of their Depression is that of dysphoria, which is present in all cases. This is a miserable sense of the pointlessness of life, from the client's viewpoint. Dysphoria can be helped with both therapy and medications. Dysphoria can be constantly present, but its intensity more likely may come and go in waves. When it comes on and stays for a while, then leaves for a while, and then returns over and over again, it appears to have a cycling nature, which some experts have classified as "Bipolar Depression." This might be more accurately described as recurring episodes of dysphoria rather than true Bipolar Depression. On the other hand, there are other clients whose recurrent waves of depression do seem to have features of mild Bipolar as well as dysphoria. There are other clients who just seem to have a low-grade chronic Depression that is not necessarily dysphoric or cyclic. And a fourth source of moodiness occurs whenever the clients might have a first date with a man; they may feel extreme giddiness and euphoria, and when the relationship fails (as it predictably may), they have extreme despair: although these are emotional up's and down's, they are in response to known environmental factors, and are not true Bipolar Depression. Regardless of the type or cycling of Depression, all these patients do need mood treatment.

Male borderlines—like men in general—are not so interested in talking about their feelings, but are much likelier to "act out" their feelings and self-treat with alcohol, drugs, and other seriously bad acting-out behaviors (petty crime, promiscuity, grifting, and so on). The males resurface periodically when they have problems with the legal system or want paperwork signed by a doctor. Occasionally, the males may voluntarily engage in therapy for a limited time if their egos have been especially badly bruised by the School of Hard Knox. Male Borderlines are typically diagnosed with narcissism, "Bipolar Depression," Borderline Disorder, Sociopathy, and/or Antisocial Behavior—they are much less likely to seek therapy voluntarily, thus we know much less about their long-term functioning. And even when they do come in for therapy, they do not stay very long. Some feminist therapists stridently denounce

Borderline Personality as a form of institutionalized misogyny invented by male psychiatrists. I think that the reality is that borderline females are in such emotional pain that they readily come in for therapy; if all the borderline males were more sensitive to their inner feelings, then they too would be likelier to come forward and talk about their painful feelings; then, we might see that a goodly amount of men also suffer this disorder, too. Additionally, a number of them probably cannot come in for appointments because they are incarcerated.

Outcome for females is not good. The predominant mood symptom is dysphoria and the main behavior is threatening to overdose. Suicide is an ever-present possibility and may be the cause of death in up to 20% of these cases. There is no cure, only treatment in the form of talk therapy, which is needed for many years. These patients usually have few or no offspring; when they do bear children, those offspring, especially the daughters, are at high risk of becoming Borderline themselves.

Outcome for borderline males: they remain about the same, and have lower suicide risk than females—although they are much likelier to be victims of violence and homicide (at the hands of other antisocial, narcissistic, or borderline males); they usually have runs-in with authority figures and the legal system; in general they like themselves the way they are. They drink and abuse drugs. They periodically feel dysphoric and come into therapy briefly until they are off on some new escapade—they do not typically announce that they are phasing out therapy: they just suddenly disappear without explanation to the therapist. Sometimes—like female borderlines—they will leave angry after-hours messages on the answering machine (while intoxicated); unlike the females, their messages may be quite menacing and allude to possible violence. With these phone calls, male borderlines effectively "self-terminate" therapy because of threats of violence. Male borderlines may pop up periodically to obtain prescriptions from (any) doctor and then disappear again. Their behaviors slow down with time. If they survive middle age, they usually turn into angry lonely old men who live on the fringes of society.

Overall outcome is not good. There is no cure. The symptoms do not improve, but rather soften with time.

COURTNEY

Courtney started to become depressed in middle school and then became more Depressed in high school. This limited some of her activities. She started to feel grousy, lousy, and miserable all the time. She started to drink any wine that was available in the household. Then she started to smoke cigarettes and then to burn herself with cigarettes. Following an overdose of Tylenol and aspirin, she was placed into the adolescent ward of a private psychiatric hospital for a month. She met two other teenage girls with similar symptoms and they became allies if not true friends. She started meeting up with them at Malls and other places, despite protests from her parents. Then she started to meet teenage boys and young men and started to tell people that she and her half-brother have ongoing sexual intimacy, a fact which he quietly denies. After she ran off to Mexico with a group of teens, her parents had her hospitalized again for two weeks, but to no avail.

One thing led to another such as petty theft (shoplifting on a dare), crashing fraternity parties at local universities, staying out all night at discotheques, (abortion), and so on. This decadence came to an abrupt halt when her family decided to send her to a cloistered girls' catholic boarding school run by stern nuns who have strict rules and uniform codes. Courtney acted out by running away, but she was apprehended and sent back to the nuns.

After graduation, she enrolled in a state university where she slept with professors, seduced young men, had an affair with her roommate, and got involved in a lot of problems. She left that university, entered another college, and eventually went on to Professional Graduate School. In her first job, she had an affair with the wife of one of her superiors, and then an affair with a top-level manager. When she was caught, she took an overdose of Benadryl at work and then called an ambulance for herself. She was back in another psychiatric hospital and was put on psychiatric disability.

Since that time, she continues to have many emotional problems and cannot maintain even a brief relationship with a man. She is not a lesbian, but participates in threesomes occasionally. She resorts to computer dating frequently, but none of those relationships pan out. She has giddiness the day before a date, and self-loathing afterwards. Men do not call her back, so she calls them. If they refuse to respond to her barrage of e-mails and phone calls, then she screams at their answering machines and resorts to vile computer "tricks." This is such a problem that it consumes half of all her therapy sessions; her therapist has had her sign many "client contracts" to limit herself to one hour per week on the computer, a rule that Courtney rarely heeds. And, she continues to act out whenever she is unhappy (dysphoric)—which may be a couple times a week. This acting-out occasionally consists of taking several pills and calling 9-1-1 to send an ambulance for an "overdose." She has a female therapist for many years who sees her weekly and fields many late night phone calls from love-sick Courtney.

She engages in regular psychotherapy sessions and is sometimes angry with her therapist, but works through it. The first time that her therapist took a vacation, Courtney took a handful of Benadryl and called an ambulance. The second time her therapist took a vacation, Courtney tried to follow. She often feels empty inside and wishes that she were dead; she sleeps too little or too much, occasionally becoming very agitated; she gains weight, takes non-prescription diet pills, and then loses too much weight. She often wishes that she were dead but then she feels gleeful because she is on permanent disability and realizes that society will take care of her for the rest of her life. She works under the table babysitting and house-sitting and then feels better when she is paid in cash. She flirts with young men at the grocery store and then flies into a silent rage when their girlfriends rush down the aisle, thinking to herself that the men were inappropriately flirting with her, after which she imagines performing violent acts on the girlfriends. This is followed by twice chanting one of her ditties such as, "all men are pigs, in this do trust, they'll fall in lust, when groins grow big, their love's a sham, so full of spam, remember this, 'cause mom knows best." Courtney may become so unnerved by her own imaginings as to have such extremes of mood as to resemble a tiny psychotic episode or a one-day manic episode.

She has a love-hate relationship with her own mother, who is also an apparent borderline. They may scream at each other on the phone and not talk for months or may nonchalantly go shopping together as if nothing had happened—and without discussing it, either.

Courtney eventually realizes that she will never find a husband in the usual way, and so she determines to get pregnant. The father of the baby, Tim, wants to be involved in the baby's life but is not interested in being involved with Courtney; instead, he suggests that his own mother rear the baby. Courtney's reaction is noted in Tim's story.

Discussion: there are a number of women with similar psychological turmoil. They may all have different modes of operation, presentation, and superficial behaviors, but the emotional problems are all about the same. Usually, they announce their presumed diagnosis as "Bipolar" and this they announce with a fair amount of pride, because they believe that this diagnosis excuses most of their behaviors ("my 'bipolar' made me do it"); some of them can become furiously resentful if [they know] their diagnosis of record is Borderline Personality Disorder, although many of them are coming to grips with the reality of this diagnosis. If they are high-functioning and understand the reality of the diagnosis, it can help them progress in therapy. Borderline females take minor overdoses, have episodes of great moodiness and occasional psychosis, and have stormy relationships with other people. Disturbed sex relations with males is a regular feature—sometimes based in reality and sometimes based on fantasy or rooted in ill-will (with the attempt to destroy the reputation of an innocent man whose only sin may have been that of rejecting her advances). These females may appear to be stalking men. Glenn Close and Michael Douglas starred in the movie, *Fatal Attraction*, which portrayed a man's run-in with a borderline female. This is a rather extreme case with a dramatized ending. Real-life situations can unfold in as many ways as there are individual personalities. For example, there was one local police case where the angry woman came to the home of her married 'boyfriend' and bit out a chunk of the man's arm muscle.

Diagnosis: Dysphoria is one of the cardinal features of this disorder. The current trend is to add a weak diagnosis of Bipolar Depression. At least 90% of the Borderline cases [who come forward for treatment] are female. Although there are male Borderlines, the men usually end up with a diagnosis of Narcissism or Antisocial Personality. The reason for this sexual difference is not clear.

Treatment: there is no FDA-approved medication for treating this disabling disorder. However, there are many possible treatments for this condition. Each treatment is prescribed "symptomatically," in other words, based on the symptoms (the same as the treatment for Secondary Depressions). Oftentimes, the Depression symptoms can be treated with a safe SSRI medication. Low-dose Zyprexa might be a good all-around medication for more severe cases of this condition, because it is FDA-approved for Bipolar disorder; Zyprexa also has pleasant anti-anxiety, anti-raging, and anti-psychotic effects. The only problem with Zyprexa is weight gain, which can be considerable; thus, Courtney must try to exercise regularly and try to avoid desserts, fast food, and junk food.

CYCLING DEPRESSION
MANIC DEPRESSION

Manic Depression is a cycling mood disorder in which people have incredibly happy moods followed by very Depressed moods. The Depression can result in suicidal thoughts. This disorder shows the greatest range of moods of all the Cycling Depressions, even more extreme than the up's and down's of Bipolar Depression. When patients like Hank are not in Depression, then they may be at baseline mood or entering into mania. Mania is characterized by hyperactivity, rapid thinking, rushed speech, euphoria, and lack of need for sleep. Mania is often followed by a phase of Depression, which can be mild, moderate, or severe. The Depression can be of very short duration or very prolonged, or anything in between. Most Manic Depressives have a specific and regular cycling pattern that they follow, and as such, each individual may have characteristic or "personalized" cycles. Some may have two separate Depressions followed by one mania and then two more Depressions. Some may have mainly manias with few Depressions or only mild Depression. Some patients who do really well on Lithium may spend prolonged periods in reasonably controlled euthymia-euphoria states during which they may rise to the top of their chosen professions (as accurately portrayed in the George Clooney movie, *Michael Clayton*). Some, however, may have an irregular and unpredictable course that does not repeat any of their previous courses of behavior, such as two hypomania episodes followed by a severe one-year suicidal Depression followed by two manias, and so on. Often, manic patients will "crash and burn" after their Mania at which time they will slump into a severe Depression. The Depression in such patients usually lasts longer than the mania, sometimes much longer. When they start to emerge from this Depression, is the precise moment at which they are likeliest to commit suicide. Suicide is a regular feature of severe Depressions in Manic Depressive illness. Some Manic Depressives have a short and mild Depression and then pop back up to their baseline state. Some Manic Depressives do not have any significant Depression phase—after "resting," they simply go back into another manic state.

Suicide is one of the commonest causes of death in Manic Depressives. Other causes come from poor self-care, accidents, and major medical illnesses. A manic is too busy to take care of himself, and a Depressive is too tired and unmotivated to go see a doctor. Accidents happen often in mania when a person is highly rushed and disorganized.

CHET

Chet grew up in LA with eccentric parents who loved to host parties at which small amounts of marijuana were enjoyed along with good wine. As he became a teenager, he likewise started to consume small amounts of wine and marijuana, but not to the point of incapacity.

The summer after he graduated from high school, he started to feel lethargic and unmotivated, and this emptiness prevented him from getting a part time job or engaging in creative activities. He entered college as a freshman, and the lethargy worsened. He could barely finish the first quarter with a "C" average and could not even finish the second quarter. He returned home and his father took him to see a family friend who was a psychiatrist.

Chet was diagnosed with a Reactive Depression due to the change from adolescence to young adulthood, high school to college, and a new set of stressors and responsibilities. Cannabis (marijuana) abuse was also a possible diagnosis. Chet was given Zoloft which did nothing for two weeks and then he seemed to develop a deeper Depression accompanied by an inner agitation. Fortunately, the psychiatrist knew the family history. One of Chet's uncles was an alcoholic, his grandmother had been addicted to narcotics, and one great uncle had died under suspicious circumstances as a young man—suicide, possibly. This information plus general observations of Chet's "eccentric" parents and unusual response to Zoloft, prompted the psychiatrist to add some bedtime Depakote. Chet continued the same treatment for another week and then one day awoke in the wee hours full of creative energy. He had a sparkling sense of humor and revealed that he had a long list of things that he needed to do. And he proceeded to try to do them all.

Within another week and a half, he became very hyperactive and rarely felt the need to sleep. He was very talkative and was so busy doing so many tasks simultaneously that he ended up accomplishing nothing. By this point, the Zoloft had already been stopped and the Depakote, increased. Over the next couple weeks, Chet narrowly escaped being hospitalized because of a number of antics such as swimming nude at a formal party. At one point he was taking the Red Line subway to Hollywood and Highland every day and was giving free tours to out-of-towners from dawn until midnight. He seemed tireless. He finally stabilized on the Depakote and needed no further antidepressant.

Discussion: Cycling Depressions can start with a Depressed phase or a non-Depressed phase. This Depression could also be just the onset of a regular Major Depression—the difference is not always apparent, but the outcomes can be very different if misdiagnosed. Chet's first episode of Manic-Depression was that of a prolonged and moderately deep Depression—it looked like a Major Depression; however, sometimes first-episode Manic-Depression can present as a Depression with a "wooden" quality (Chet's emotional state resembles that of a piece of timber). These episodes can persist for a long time unless treated. If Depression is the first episode of Manic Depression, then treatment must be administered carefully. An antidepressant can launch a person like Chet into mania. (But if Chet simply had had a Major Depression, then an anti-mania mood stabilizer drug could have Depressed him further.) In the days before medications, these Manic-Depression Depressions could be very serious, prolonged, and associated with suicide attempts. In Chet's case, the Depression was deep enough that he spent three weeks on an antidepressant before having any apparent response: and the response was undesirable because it launched him into a mild mania (a Manic Depressive who is at baseline, neither Depressed nor manic, can be launched into mania by antidepressants in a few short days).

So how do we provide the best treatment? In other words, how do we know that a first-time Depression is Manic Depression and not just ordinary Depression? We may not, but hopefully we determine this by analyzing other data. First, Chet has a family history suggestive of mood disorders and alcoholism. Statistically, this puts him at added risk of having Manic Depression possibly due to his "genetics." Secondly, his delayed response to an antidepressant is not typical of a person with mild Depression. Most people with a mild Major Depression will have certain predictable side-effects in the first week* then start to feel calmer but motivated within a week or two. Some people with a moderate Major Depression may take the medication for four to six weeks and have little response (like Chet), but they will not become manic. Even more confusing, some Major Depression patients can quickly become hypomanic from an antidepressant. They, however, are not Manic Depressive if the mania disappears the day after stopping the medication. These patients are just exquisitely sensitive to certain antidepressants.** The easiest maneuver in these cases is to switch to another antidepressant to treat the Major Depression—these patients will not have a paradoxical hypomania from every antidepressant (unlike manic-depressives who will be launched into mania by any/all antidepressants).

Diagnosis: Manic Depression, first episode Depressed; requires standard anti-mania medications to maintain baseline behavior.

Treatment: Depakote 1000 mg; avoid drugs and alcohol which may trigger mania or increase the risk of another cycling mood episode. Street drugs and alcohol can cause cycling by any of several mechanisms: interfering with the Depakote effect, de-stabilizing Chet's nervous system, disinhibiting him (decreasing his cautiousness), or jeopardizing his judgment by "telling" him that he is not Manic Depressive. Once Chet is under the influence of drugs, he will lose control and start to abuse drugs and alcohol, which results in a downward emotional spiral.

Outcome: Chet no longer uses marijuana and is enrolled in one of the best automotive design schools on the West Coast. He will probably have this cycling mood disorder for life. Whether it needs to be medicated continuously remains to be seen, but that is most advisable.

---

*each antidepressant has its own characteristic first-week side effects—any deviant side effects can be a clue that treatment is off-track
**They can be stabilized successfully on that same antidepressant if they are restarted on very tiny doses of it, after which the doses can be raised by tiny amounts over the next few months. Then they should be

able to tolerate typical adult doses. The real difficulty in these cases is dividing the medication into appropriately tiny doses, which may require resorting to the use of liquid medication or quartering tablets (and placing the fragment into an empty gelatin capsule to slow absorption). Prozac is notorious for causing this odd reaction in Dysthymia and Major Depression.

HANK

Hank was an eldest son and came from modest circumstances: his father was a plumber. Hank had lost his mother to breast cancer when he was sixteen. Hank helped raise his younger siblings because his father worked long hours and was also on-call for plumbing emergencies. Hank had been an exceptional student throughout high school and cared for his mother during her prolonged illness. For this reason, he continued to live at home while working his way through a local state college. He passed his real estate exam and became very successful at that endeavor. He was named top realtor in his firm, a notable "first" for someone so young.

He earned enough money to subsidize college educations for his younger siblings. During this time, he had "launched" into a state of great joy, productivity, and energy, showing decreased need for sleep. He was busy all the time showing homes, conducting business, and responding to his cell phone at all hours. This high level of commitment continued for a few years after which he went into an emotional slump, and his activity levels decreased. He felt mentally fatigued, and his motivation decreased to a point where his functioning was barely mediocre. He found time to develop introspective interests and solo activities such as running and hiking with his dog. During this time, he met Gaile, and they started a long-term relationship. Within a year and a half, he had proposed to her. Once again, he began to feel "supercharged" and launched back into the real estate business with renewed vigor and gusto, making many sales and achieving much financial success. He married Gaile. This flurry of activity continued, and he was still able to allot time to Gaile, primarily because he did not need more than five hours sleep.

Around this time, he started to make some errors in contracts and to exhibit some changes in his behavior. He was over-talkative, sleeping little, showing questionable judgment, and spending more money. He seemed to be running around in circles with one foot nailed to the floor. The real estate firm decided to "downsize," as a result of which he went out on his own and started his own real estate company that did well.

Nine months later, he went through another period of slow activity and found renewed time to spend watching movies quietly with his wife and baby son on the weekends. He also found time to go back to weekend school and enroll in an MBA program.

After this, he became active again for a year, then very active for that next year, after which he became quite manic, making many mistakes in his business. His real estate license was in jeopardy. During this time, he ended up in the psychiatric emergency room and was involuntarily sent to a psychiatric hospital where the doctor and his wife both agreed that he needed Lithium. Hank discovered that Lithium acted as a "governor" on his "high-flying" tendencies without having an adverse effect on his ability to conduct business. He quickly finished his MBA degree that was awarded "with distinction," and he continued to do well on Lithium for almost three decades until it started to cause him some decreased kidney function.

Discussion: this is a classic case of Manic Depression in which the patient never really has profound Depressions—or, his Depressions manifest as "slow" times in his life that do not plague him with the burden of a crippling Depression. Many of these cases are of successful men who have always been charismatic, popular, tireless, and outgoing overachievers since they were children. Some of them may abuse alcohol, but more often, they appear as a class of "workaholics." They usually take the same dose of fairly high-dose Lithium year after year without need to change it or add extra medications. They remain stable for decades. The biggest hurdle in their lives may occur when they are older and they must quit taking Lithium because of its long-term side effects (early kidney problems and sluggish thyroid gland).

In cases like Hank's, Lithium acts to stabilize mood; to a lesser degree, it may prevent recurrent Depressions.

These patients usually have some family history of Mood Disorders or Depressive-Equivalent Disorders. Hank's mother's mother, in this case, was a highly accomplished woman who also became addicted to over-the-counter opium elixir until her access was cut off by the Harrison Drug Act.

Diagnosis: Manic Depression (also called Bipolar I)

Rx: Lithium 1200 mg a day for the next twenty-some years until his kidney functions started to decrease, whereupon he was changed to Depakote.

Outcome: Hank continued to take Lithium for many years and was a successful and respected businessman in his community (George Clooney starred in the movie, *Michael Clayton*, in which he helped such a man as Hank.) Hank was active in many community organizations, and had three sons, one of whom developed an episode of Major Depression as a teenager (that later turned into Recurrent Unipolar Depression—this is his genetic legacy from Hank). Another son became a successful (but alcoholic) land developer-realtor-businessman (male alcoholism is common in families with serious mood disorders). The youngest son chose to work in plumbing with his grandfather, Hank's father.

Suicide is much less of a serious problem in cases like Hank's since these types of Manic Depressives rarely become severely Depressed and also since the Lithium typically prevents them from having serious recurrent Depressions; however, the risk of suicide is ever-present in all cycling mood disorders and can definitely increase in the elderly Manic Depressive population, regardless of earlier adult cycling patterns. Some of these men may have a defining episode later in life in which the lithium is no longer helpful, or they have a serious episode ("nervous breakdown") when they try to change from lithium to Depakote. Alcohol consumption can sometimes figure into the equation later in life. Alcohol abuse can increase in the retirement years and lead to Depression and suicidal tendencies.

CYCLING DEPRESSION
CYCLOTHYMIA

This is a third "flavor" of Cycling Depression and it is also the mildest form. In Cyclothymia, episodes of dysthymia (low moods) alternate cyclically with episodes of non-Depression. The episodes of non-Depression may consist of euthymia (a state of feeling quite content and satisfied), euphoria (joyousness), or even mild hypomania. The appearance of euthymia or euphoria may occur in the same person for different episodes of non-Depression. In other words, Cyclothymia is like a mild Bipolar Depression. Cyclothymic patients have periods of mildly happy moods followed by periods of mildly unhappy or absolutely dismal moods.

Euthymia refers to a feeling of well-being. Euthymia is the goal for which we strive in treatment of all Depressions, especially cycling Depressions. Sometimes it can be achieved by use of medications, and sometimes we can approach it but never arrive. There is more on this topic above in the introduction to Cycling Depressions.

RAJ (RAJACHANDRA)
He had been a good science student in high school, and graduated early, after which he went to college in Chicago.

In the Fall semester of his freshman year, soon after arriving at college, he started to feel a loss of motivation. His grades did not fall very much at all, but he needed more time to do his homework, which seemed to cut into any recreational time. This was despite the fact that he felt enthusiastic about his coursework. Then he met a girl from India, Madhu, who was a sophomore in his college. They both seemed very compatible and comfortable with each other. His parents were thrilled. However, family crisis forced Madhu to leave college after the first semester. Raj also began to suspect that his roommate was prejudiced against non-Europeans; Raj heard through the grapevine that his roommate was applying for a new roommate in spring semester. All of these events seemed to be slowly grinding away at Raj's motivation and luster.

When Raj returned to L.A. for winter break, his mother was concerned by his apparent loss of spark and eagerness. Raj talked with his parents and after some resistance, they were able to convince him to start appointments with the counseling service when he returned to college after winter break.

So, Raj engaged in psychotherapy and counseling at the college and seemed to have much improvement. He was lively, energetic, and took extra classes, and made excellent grades. Madhu returned to college after the family crisis and Raj was feeling jubilant. He threw himself into the relationship and into scholastics and earned a 4.0 GPA for that semester. All went well until the next semester when he seemed to become very withdrawn and unmotivated again for no apparent reason—nothing had changed except for his mood. Raj returned to the school counseling services, and it was decided to start Raj on Lexapro. And he improved. Then he shifted back into a highly activated mood and felt thrilled by life, although he was not at any time truly out of control or bizarre—he was simply possessed by uncommonly good joyousness and optimism. Trileptal was added in low doses and he began to feel "perfected." He continued to take medication and extra classes and finished his B.S. and M.S. At times, he had felt a little slowed, but it was not disabling and not too long lasting. Raj attempted to quit the medications with the result that he had another Depression followed by "irrational silliness" as Madhu called it. He resumed his medications. He later married Madhu and held down a good job.

Discussion: Raj has developed a tendency to have low-grade Depressions interspersed with episodes of over-exuberance. This is called Cyclothymia which consists of periods of Dysthymia followed by periods of very happy moods. This can be treated with low doses of an antidepressant (such as Lexapro) plus equally low doses of a mild mood stabilizer or sedating antidepressant, Trileptal, in this case.

Diagnosis: Cyclothymia

Rx: Lexapro 7½ mg and Trileptal 225 mg.

Outcome: good to very good

CYCLING DEPRESSION

RECURRENT UNIPOLAR DEPRESSION (RUPD)

A person who has experienced an episode of Major Depression may not become Depressed again later in life. However, it is possible that he could have a second Depressive episode, such as Reactive Depression, Secondary Depression, or a repeat episode of Major Depression. He might also be likely much later in life to develop Alzheimer's Depression or other psychiatric conditions (psychosis or anxiety).

If a person does have a second episode of Major Depression that clears up with treatment after a year or two, then it may not ever come back. If it comes back for a third time and starts to recur in a cyclical pattern and meets certain other requirements, then it may actually be a type of Major Depression that is coming in cycles, called Recurrent Unipolar Depression (RUPD). In hindsight, the first episode of Major Depression was the first cycle of RUPD, and the second episode of Major Depression was the second cycle of RUPD. Thus, RUPD feels like Major Depression but occurs twice or more.

RUPD is a form of Cycling Mood Disorder that has the symptoms of Major Depression, but it may require slightly different treatment. Its cycling nature may respond well to low doses of certain mood stabilizers that are useful in the treatment of Cycling Depressions such as Lithium, Lamictal, Trileptal, and Depakote (response to Tegretol is less likely). By "respond well", I mean that these mood stabilizers should stop it from cycling. The mood stabilizers will not treat the Depression. The Depression will still require the use of an antidepressant. Thus, the patient may end up taking a mood stabilizer and an antidepressant.

141

Often there is some family history of Cycling Mood Disorders as well as a family history of "Depression-Equivalent Disorders," such as ADHD and compulsive disorders, notably alcoholism. Furthermore, the cycling of RUPD should resemble the cycling of Cyclothymia, Bipolar, or Manic Depression. This is not to say that the cycling is regular like the seasons of the year, but that it is "irregularly regular" in the same ways that the other Cycling Moods cycle. In RUPD, unlike the other mood disorders, the "up" phase is just baseline behavior or euthymia.

The observant reader may also want to know what is the difference between Chronic Depression and RUPD: Chronic Depressive does not cycle. Its Depressive symptoms tend to persist and remain the same, month after month, year after year; and, the patient usually has a sense of the continuing presence of the underlying Depression, whereas the RUPD patient can actually return to near-baseline functioning (perhaps 85% or better). However, Chronic Depressives can sometimes rise up to feel 65-85% better, too, if the right medications are found. Chronic Depressives usually take the same dose of the same medicine for years, whereas RUPD patients may need to adjust dosage depending upon their cycle.

BARNEY

Barney's mother became a late-life alcoholic and his father was always a heavy social drinker. Barney's first episode of Depression occurred rather early in life. This first Depressive episode occurred before most modern antidepressants existed; however, ECT (Shock Treatments) had been very effective back then, and he had a near-complete recovery. A second episode occurred a couple years later and was treated with talk therapy. A year later he had a third episode of Depression for which he received a second course of ECT and the third episode did clear within three weeks, allowing him to get back to work without a lengthy leave of absence. Although he had a few residual symptoms, he did well for several years, possibly because he was having the best time of his life, professionally and personally. Then he became Depressed again, and was given Nardil which worked well for several years. Then he felt that his body was "rejecting" the medication, so he and his doctor decided to stop it. Within a year, he became Depressed again and tried Norpramin which helped him to feel much better. He continued that medication at a fairly high dose for years. When he started to have Norpramin side effects and new symptoms of guilt, his doctor changed him to Triavil; Barney felt well for nine years until his hands started shaking uncontrollably. Meanwhile his psychiatrist had learned more about RUPD and modified Barney's diagnosis. The Trilafon was stopped and the doctor added low dose Lithium and Elavil. Barney did quite well for a few months, and then became very tired so that the Lithium dose was taken down to very low levels. After this, Barney did quite well. Then that combination seemed to lose its effect and he was also developing a number of medication side effects (partly due to his age), so Lithium was replaced with Lamictal. Further side effects occurred from aging, and the Elavil was replaced with high-dose Lexapro. Barney has remained stable to date.

Discussion: the first important fact is that Barney's first and third episodes of Depression responded well to ECT. ECT is usually reserved for very serious Depressions which respond quite well to it (Cycling Depressions might be more serious than Major Depression); however, since there were so few treatment options available back then, ECT was used more often: for severe and moderate Depressions, for Major Depression and Cycling Depression. We cannot know the exact type of Barney's Depression just by hindsight. But we do now know that ECT yields superior results in serious conditions, and is not so effective for less serious Depressions; so we can infer that his Depression was serious and probably severe. As his story unfolds, new facts pop up such as the tendency of his Depression to cycle, and of the cycles to become more frequent and harder to treat. He also responds well to the addition of mood stabilizers (not a regular treatment tactic in Major Depression). Additionally, he has a family history for alcoholism, which can be a clue to a Cycling Depression. As far as personal history, Barney did have the compulsive trait of being a "work-a-holic" which can be a compulsive trait found in Manic Depression as well as in alcoholic families and families with Depression-equivalent disorders.

Diagnosis: RUPD: Recurrent Unipolar Depression.

Treatment: continue Lexapro and Lamictal.

Outcome: he will need continuous medication treatment indefinitely, and he will probably need at least two mood medications.

•

OTHER DEPRESSIONS

GRIEF WITH DEPRESSION (PROLONGED GRIEF)

Psychiatrists usually do not consider grief to be a psychiatric diagnosis since it is a normal part of our life experience. Depressive symptoms such as sadness, weeping, and social withdrawal are completely normal symptoms after the loss of a loved one. Loss of appetite or loss of weight may be very common in grief but usually begin to improve after a few months. Normal recovery involves sadness (depression), concern for the deceased, adjusting to the absence of the loved one, learning to adjust to the sudden onset of this new phase of life for the survivor, and then dealing with it effectively. Normally, grief will slowly improve over a number of months or years, and the grief-stricken person can move on with his life. However, in some cases, the period of depression (sadness) continues without improvement (no return to baseline) and then merges into Minor Depression (or one of the other forms of Depression). Minor Depression may become a prolonged grief, which either stays the same indefinitely or improves spontaneously after a couple years. However, Minor Depression can deteriorate further into one of the major Depressions. Treating the Minor Depression promptly may prevent its further deterioration into one of the major Depressions, or the Minor Depression may progress even if it does receive timely treatment, based on the type of Depression that is present. This is unfortunate, but fortunately, modern treatments are available and usually beneficial.

ALTAGRACIA (NICKNAME: TATA)

Tata is from Santo Domingo and comes from a genteel but poor family. She met and married Juan Carlos, a Mexican-American, who had been stationed in Santo Domingo. They fell in love at first sight and before he went back to Los Angeles, he and Tata were married. They had three children and lived a middle-class life on the west side of Los Angeles. Juan Carlos had a good job, which afforded him a pension. Unfortunately, he passed away two years after taking early retirement.

Altagracia had learned English fairly well, but always had a yearning for her hometown, which seemed so far away. She often returned there with her children to spend a long summer vacation with her extended family and friends.

After the death of her husband, she did develop sadness from grief, but also became extremely anxious about her future without him because she had depended so much on him. This was the first time that she had such prolonged anxiety. After her husband's death, she often visited her family doctor, Dr. Sanchez, to tell him about her anxiety, her anxious stomach, her headaches, insomnia, backache, and so on (see "somatizing" in the Vocabulary). Eventually, he tells her that she has "*nervios*" (a nervous and anxious Depression) and prescribes her Ativan, which is a minor tranquilizer and not an antidepressant. The end result is that she starts to take a minor tranquilizer to treat her grief, sadness, and anxiety, the symptoms of which collectively merge and emerge as an Anxious Depression.

Ativan is a habit-forming drug in the Valium family and will not help grief or Depression. On the contrary, it is a "downer." Tata—like many patients—will continue to raise the dose of Ativan in the elusive hope that it will help her grief and Depression. The end result is that she is taking more Ativan than prescribed and actually feels worse than before starting it. She has gone from one half milligram Ativan a day to one milligram four times a day, an eight-fold increase. She becomes more Depressed and is now becoming addicted to Ativan. Then she starts to wake up every morning with anxiety which is due to Ativan withdrawal. If more than six or eight hours pass, she will start to have Ativan withdrawal and will feel very anxious. She is unaware that this is withdrawal and interprets it as the original anxiety, which, therefore, requires a higher dose. Thus, she increases the Ativan several times more on her own and without any input from Dr. Sanchez. All this while, she still has the underlying Depression that has also not been treated. She will eventually have a panic attack from Ativan withdrawal, which she thinks is a heart attack (symptoms can be similar) and takes an ambulance ride to the nearest Emergency Room (ER). While in the ER, she is given enough Ativan to calm her down and is later released into the care of one of her adult children. The ER staff treats the immediate problem (Ativan withdrawal) but cannot treat long-term problems, such as ongoing Depression—this type of problem is usually treated by her family doctor or a psychiatrist.

Eventually she will be sent to a psychiatrist, Dr. Ps, who starts treatment for Depression. Dr. Ps may—or may not—be successful at weaning her off Ativan totally. Unfortunately, the Ativan makes her Depression more difficult to treat because Ativan is a depressant of the nervous system and causes a Secondary Depression ("Depression due to Ativan").

Discussion: many of these patients like Tata start out with Anxiety Reaction or an Anxious Depression. Then Tata becomes addicted to a drug like Ativan (or Xanax or Valium). The Ativan then becomes a second source of Depression, a Secondary Depression. Even worse, once Tata becomes addicted to Ativan, she often does not respond well to standard antidepressants, such as Paxil (and other SSRI's). All she wants is more drug (Ativan) with the same effect—not different medications like Paxil that have different effects. When patients like Tata first start on antidepressants like Paxil for Anxious Depression, the Paxil will not control the anxiety for at least two to eight weeks. Tata, therefore, will need to continue the Ativan during this time, which only progresses the Ativan addiction for a couple more months. Furthermore, if the antidepressant causes the slightest side effects in the first two weeks of treatment (as often happens), then patients like Tata will immediately stop the antidepressant and refuse to try any more antidepressants. In general, patients like Tata, when exposed first-time to a standard antidepressant, will feel anxiety side effects during the first two weeks of treatment—this can be a normal side effect of Paxil (and SSRI's). This is why I start these patients on tiny amounts of Paxil in the beginning of treatment. The first day upon which Paxil causes anxiety, these patients will refuse to take any more, stating that it makes them more anxious (it worsens their Anxious Depression). So they end up with two sources of Depression and three sources of anxiety which feed into each other over and over again. The two sources of Depression are prolonged grief and Ativan; the three sources of anxiety are Anxious Depression, initial stimulating effects of Paxil, and Ativan withdrawal (impending Ativan withdrawal as each dose wears off).

Diagnosis: Grief and Anxious Depression

Treatment: There are **three choices**, depending on whether Tata has **more Depression** than anxiety, **more anxiety** than Depression, or **equal amounts** of both. In the first case, of **more Depression**, Tata starts on a sedating and calmative antidepressant (Remeron or Trazodone at bedtime; or Norpramin or Pamelor 10 mg thrice daily) and then tries to reduce the Ativan dosage slowly throughout the daytime. Sedating antidepressants may be effective, but once again, patients like Tata will have sedating side effects for the first week(s); these side effects may not seem pleasant until the full antidepressant effect takes hold. These sedating effects will not be the same as those of Ativan, but will gradually become more pleasing after a few months. In the second case, patients with **more anxiety** can sometimes be weaned off Ativan by using one of the mood stabilizers: Zyprexa and Depakote work very well in this regard. The mood stabilizer may continue as the primary treatment. Patients with about **equal amounts** of Depression and anxiety are ideal candidates for a switch to Paxil-like medications as outlined in the Discussion paragraph above. One thing is certain: Tata will never feel really good again while she is on this daily cycle of mild Ativan intoxication and withdrawal.

Outcome: is poor to fair if she stays home alone and does not socialize with other widows and seniors; Outcome is much better if she can treat the Depression and anxiety with non-addicting medications and then go out to socialize regularly with friends and family and develop a hobby (if she does not already have one) such as gardening or knitting.

ENRIQUE

He has recently been widowed and lives alone now. Two of his adult children live very nearby, and two others live in greater Los Angeles. He feels sad and misses his wife of forty-five years and has stopped attending any social functions, including church. He feels lonely, and also tries to shun family events, but his adult children will not let him retreat into total self-isolation. They realize that his depression is becoming a Depression. His daughter takes him to see his family doctor, Dr. Sanchez, who gives him Lexapro. Enrique does not like that medicine because of its initial side effects (anxiety, upset stomach) and quits taking it. He continues to see Dr. Sanchez for frequent complaints of backache, loss of appetite, poor sleep, and weird dreams (see "somatizing" in the Vocabulary). Dr. Sanchez prescribes him Zoloft and then Paxil, both to no avail. Enrique reaches a stalemate with Dr. Sanchez who suggests that Enrique's daughter take him to see the staff psychiatrist, Dr. Ps, who diagnoses Enrique with a prolonged grief that is merging into a minor Depression. He is given Remeron but does not want to take that either. He refuses to go back to see the psychiatrist. He continues to mope around the house for several months more, and at this time, two of his sons provide "strong encouragement" and bring him back to Dr. Ps to try yet another medication (Wellbutrin-SR). Enrique digs in his heels saying that he is in mourning but is not Depressed and does not want to see psychiatrists. He says that his feelings are "normal." The family disagrees and cites evidence that he is deteriorating further. More "discussion" takes place during which he reminds them that they cannot possibly know what he is feeling. Ultimately, Enrique is prescribed Prozac-Weekly. His whole family continues to have family Sundays in Enrique's home. On these occasions, his three adult sons quietly take him into his bedroom, shut the door, and insist that he take one Prozac-Weekly pill, which he grudgingly does. They check his mouth to verify that he is not "cheeking" the pill (to prevent his hiding it in his cheek and then spitting it out later). After a few months, Enrique stabilizes somewhat, and is not so symptomatic as before.

Diagnosis: Minor Depression, resulting from prolonged grief

Rx: one capsule of Prozac-Weekly-90 mg to be taken every Sunday; Prozac is not a first-line or second-line medication in the older population, but in this case it needs to be.

Outcome: his Depression did improve somewhat. He agreed to let his daughter drop him off twice a week at Senior Center where he did some socializing. He also attended grief group there. He resumed attending mass once a week, and usually looked forward to family

Sunday at his house. His sons still had to supervise his pill-taking. With all these measures in place, he had between 35-50% improvement. If he had been willing to admit his Depression, try different medicines, and follow all other treatment guidelines, he could have had well over 50% improvement. In some of these bereavement cases, the surviving spouse has only a modest improvement, at best. But sometimes, something is better than nothing. Cases like this amply demonstrate how catastrophic death can be for the surviving spouse.

POST-PARTUM DEPRESSION

(also, see Topic on Pregnancy at end of Part Three)
In Latin, "post-partum" means "after giving birth"

This is a Depression/depression occurring after a baby is born. In its mildest form, it is called "baby blues," which can be quite common, but is almost never so significant as to require psychiatric treatment. It is a Minor Depression that is usually treated by the obstetrician or family doctor. If the "baby blues" become more serious, the new mother can develop a mild Major Depression, called Post-partum Depression. This may be treated by the family doctor or obstetrician. The big difference, practically speaking, between "baby blues" and Post-partum Depression is that the new mother who has a clinical Depression might stop bonding with the baby. In mild cases, she will regret the loss of her earlier carefree days when she imagined herself prettier and more desirable. The baby may be viewed as an intervening factor that has permanently altered her. In these cases, the mother needs a mild antidepressant. She cannot go on breast-feeding because psychiatric medications pass into the breast milk and then into the baby. Additionally, she needs to have twenty-four hour supervision until the antidepressant starts to lift her spirits to the point where she feels renewed joy of motherhood (within two months, hopefully). This supervision is often basically provided by her husband at night and her relatives in the daytime (sister, mother, mother-in-law, nanny).

Apart from the mild cases, which account for most cases, Post-partum Depression may also become moderate, severe, or severely psychotic. Moderate Post-partum Depression is less common than mild Depression, and severe Depression is rarer yet. Severe psychotic cases are very rare and are often viewed on the six o'clock news because felonies are involved. Such felonies include kidnapping, reckless endangerment, child (infant) abuse, suicide, homicide, filicide (killing of the infant and other offspring), and so on. These cases are sensational. Fortunately, they are very rare. Such cases can become so bad that the new mother falls into a Psychotic Depression which is the prime time when a new mother will kill the baby and try to kill herself too. This is her reasoning: her psychosis tells her that the world is a horrible place. She believes that she would be better off dead. She does not want to abandon the baby to such a horrible world without its mother, so she feels obligated to take it with her. Or, she may hear voices telling her to come to heaven. And she wants to be united in heaven with the baby who will have a much better life [up] there. Psychosis is not rational. A mild Depression may become moderate which may become severe. Any doctor, who presumes to treat post-partum Depression, should be aware of these possibilities.

Cases of moderate post-partum Depression require aggressive treatment and may require hospitalization. At the very least, major medications will be involved and strict supervision will be needed around the clock. In severe cases, the mother is totally unable to care for the baby and provisions should be made. Major medications will be needed and hospitalization may be necessary (to protect her and the infant from herself). Mild cases may respond well to a mild antidepressant within a few weeks; and, moderate cases, within a couple months. Severe cases may require many months, and the mother may never be mentally quite the same again. Ever. The aftermath of severe psychotic cases is completely unpredictable, even with prolonged and aggressive treatment.

Anti-depressants and other psychiatric drugs pass through breast milk. The baby may not have breast milk. Once a woman has had Post-partum Depression, she is at risk for having it return with all following pregnancies. And if it does return, it might be worse in the following episodes. Her sisters also may be at high risk of this type of Depression.

CECILE

Here is an example of a major romantic disappointment: Cecile is a young lady who became romantically involved with Bert, her unmarried boss, who was only a year older than she. After putting up with his erratic behaviors, she came to believe that he had a possible drinking problem. Worse than that, she learned that he was engaged to someone who lived in San Diego. She had trouble saying "no" to him. She thought that she loved him. He told her that he was going to break up with his fiancée, but did not know how to do that long-distance and he wanted to see where the relationship with Cecile was leading him.

Cecile became frustrated, then disappointed, and then felt depressed. She continued to obsess about Bert: where he was, what he was doing, and with whom he was doing it. Their relationship had been going on for almost a year. She had some of the most memorable moments in her adult life with Bert, but also some low points. Sometimes he would not show up, or if he did he was either giddy and euphoric or tipsy. Once he passed out in Oldtown Pasadena and was rushed to the nearby ER.

Cecile started to feel sluggish and unresponsive and she began to self-isolate. She lost her appetite but gained weight. She woke up late every morning feeling "half-way normal", but as the day wore on she became disheartened and sluggish. In the evening she would develop a feeling of dread, and then felt very miserable at night and could not sleep. All her symptoms felt worse at night. She started to wonder if she would need to buy "plus-size" clothes some day and then began to obsess about that, too. (But that never came to pass.) She discussed this with her mother who came from a family where half the men were alcoholics. Her mother suggested that Cecile see a therapist and attend Alanon meetings.

Cecile commenced therapy with a therapist who then sent her to see the supervising psychiatrist who started her on Prozac. Cecile started to feel better. Within a couple weeks, she was feeling joyous—partly because Bert had asked her to marry him. They were married, she continued the Prozac, and he started showing up sporadically at AA meetings, trying to quit. Nothing more was said of "San Diego." After a year, she quit the Prozac and was feeling stable. Bert's drinking had decreased to about one weekend binge per month. When Cecile unexpectedly became pregnant, Bert started drinking heavily and ended up spending one whole weekend in San Diego, although he was apparently passed out the whole weekend—but he was still in *that woman's* apartment, as Cecile later found out. Bert was not present for the days before, during and after the baby was born. Cecile gave birth alone and almost immediately started to become Depressed. She began to regret the last two years of her life. She went to see her family doctor who gave her a one-month supply of Prozac, told her not to breastfeed, and sent her back to the psychiatrist who continued the Prozac and also told her not to breastfeed as Prozac would be in the milk. She felt better with the medication, but nothing could erase her heartache.

Cecile divorced Bert a few years later, and she eventually managed to find a healing environment in Alanon.

Discussion: women from alcoholic families tend—more often than not—to choose alcoholic husbands. Cecile had a Depression at the end of the first year of her relationship with Bert, which is not a good sign. Then she had a positive reaction to the marriage proposal. This is a reactive euphoria and does not mean that the Depression is over, by any means. This emotional outpouring should not be confused with true happiness. Then she developed a mild Post-partum Depression that responded well to her original antidepressant (not at all uncommon). She had a typical experience with an alcoholic husband, and decided for her own sanity to bail out of the relationship, a difficult decision. Prozac is safe enough in pregnancy but should be avoided if breastfeeding.

Diagnosis: mild Major Depression, co-dependence, and Post-partum Depression.

Treatment: Alanon and Prozac.

Outcome: good if she follows through with appropriate treatment; otherwise, fair to poor. As a result of the first Post-partum Depression, she is now at increased risk for Post-partum Depression after any future pregnancies: the Post-partum Depression can get worse with each pregnancy.

JANICE

She is thirty-two years old and had her first baby seven months ago. She has noted recently that she feels sluggish and unmotivated. She is so tired and un-reactive that her husband usually has to take care of the baby in the wee hours. She is gaining weight, losing some hair, and feeling tired. Her family doctor orders some lab tests; then he sends her to Dr. Ps, a psychiatrist who treats her with Prozac for a month, but she is not responding as expected. The Prozac is increased, and Janice comes back in three weeks. She now mentions the weight gain and loss of hair; by now, her hair loss has worsened, her hair has become dry and frazzled, and she has lost part of her eyebrows. Dr. Ps then pores over her lab tests and discovers that the lab had rejected her recent thyroid test for being in the wrong test tube. Dr. Ps re-orders the thyroid test which reveals a low thyroid function. She is sent back to her family doctor for thyroid treatment. A month later, she is feeling "normal" when she returns to see Dr. Ps, so together they decide to stop the Prozac, after which she feels fine. (this is from a real case)

Discussion: She acquired a secondary Depression caused by hypothyroidism ("low thyroid function"). And the "low thyroid" was related to childbirth (not uncommon). This chain of medical events happens. Psychiatrists do see new mothers with a number of types of Depressions, some of which are considered purely psychiatric ("Post-partum Depression"). In truth, the chemical and physiological changes during pregnancy probably qualify many of the so-called "psychiatric" causes of post-partum Depression to be medical—due to hormonal alterations in pregnancy. We still have not identified the causes and treatments of these. Janice has a physical Depression that affects the physical organ of the brain; when the brain slows down, Janice feels a secondary mental Depression. This is another way that psychiatry differs from all other medical specialties: the physical organ involved in the specialty is also involved in generating and interpreting all the symptoms of that disease; the physical organ also affects the patient's perception of his special disease. This does not happen, for example, in cardiology or dermatology. The heart (or skin) cannot act upon itself to modify, mollify, mask, mimic, or misinterpret its symptoms or its actual disease state.

Diagnosis: Secondary Depression due to Low Thyroid (Hypothyroidism)

Treatment: thyroid hormone is supplied by her family doctor; she does not need to see a psychiatrist (at this time).

Outcome: excellent. Becoming Depressed from low thyroid hormone levels in the post-partum period does not make her a psychiatric patient or suggest that she ever will be.

OTHER DEPRESSION: WINTER DEPRESSION

(see stories of Meg and Clairice)

In northern climates, the winters are longer and colder. People—like animals—tend to change biochemically in response to the cold. This is a hibernation reflex which is apparently normal. Winter Depression symptoms are those of hibernation reflex: gaining weight by eating extra carbohydrates, sleeping longer and more deeply, feeling less motivated, and feeling withdrawn. Some people become sensitive to these symptoms, especially the withdrawal. In comparison to their summer activities which they would rate as zero or neutral, their winter withdrawal feels like a negative state, that presents as Depression symptoms. This is why people seek treatment against the feelings of the hibernation reflex. Light-boxes which produce natural sunlight (full spectrum light) can be quite helpful. Light-boxes provide excellent treatment of winter Depression without the need to take pills. Winter Depression is also called SAD (Seasonal Affective Disorder). The risk of Winter Depression is increased in gloomier climates and in the northernmost latitudes. Some experts report that rates of alcoholism increase as the latitude increases, which may represent an attempt at self-treatment. Alcohol will not cure SAD. There are rare cases of SAD occurring not in the winter, but rather during summer.

SECONDARY DEPRESSIONS

Secondary Depression is a Depression due to a known cause, such as a medical disorder or chemicals. The known causes may be outside the patient's control—or within his control. In such cases, the disease or chemical is considered the primary disorder (known cause) and the Secondary Depression is a secondary disorder; thus, the Depression is secondary to the primary cause. Secondary Depression is often outside the patient's control, as in the case of medical diseases or life-saving treatments that the patient must take in order to survive the medical disease. On the other hand, sometimes the cause is within the patient's control. He might be doing something toxic to himself or refusing to do something beneficial for himself. Toxic behaviors that he does to himself would be drinking and drugging (or any other self-destructive compulsive behavior). Refusal of self-care can lead to a Secondary Depression also and is within the patient's control. If a person refuses to do something healthful to stave off Depression—or purposely avoids doing something to prevent Depression—then that could also be a Secondary Depression. Examples are: refusing to take insulin or AIDS medicines, avoiding AA meetings, skipping therapy sessions, refusal to buy thyroid pills (see Janice's story above), and so on.

Secondary Depression caused by a known medical disorder is caused biochemically by a medical disease, which is known to cause Depression as part of the disease process. Such diseases include certain medical disorders, neurological disorders, and certain (other) psychiatric disorders. Medical disorders may involve hormonal imbalances (thyroid gland, pituitary gland, or adrenal gland). Correcting the hormonal imbalance should correct the Depression. Sometimes the medical disorder does not cause Depression, but the treatment for the medical disorder

156

causes Secondary Depression. For example, hepatitis-C does not cause a major Depression, but the treatment for Hepatitis-C (Interferon) causes serious Depression in many patients. Many neurological diseases can cause Depression, because neurological disease is a disease of the brain. And any disease that damages the brain can result in a Depressed brain: Multiple Sclerosis, Alzheimer's, and Parkinsonism can cause Secondary Depression. As far as psychiatric disorders, chronic anxiety patients who suffer long enough from an untreated anxiety disorder can develop a Secondary Depression: by the time, they come to a psychiatrist, they will then have two problems: primary anxiety plus Secondary Depression. Sometimes schizophrenic patients can develop a temporary Depression after a psychotic "break-down." PTSD is a severe anxiety disorder that may have a component of Secondary Depression.

However, there are patients who have a reactive Depression to a new medical diagnosis. If a person becomes Depressed when he is told that he has new-onset diabetes, then he is having a Reactive Depression, a reaction to bad news. This is not a Secondary Depression, because the actual disease of diabetes is not known to cause secondary Depression directly on a biochemical basis.

As far as chemicals, various chemicals can cause Depression. In every major class and family of chemicals, there are always a couple members in that family or class capable of causing Depression. Certain prescription medications can cause Depression. Among the blood pressure pills, Inderal causes a serious Depression. Among the stomach pills, Reglan and Tagamet can cause Depression. Also, Prednisone, Chantix, and others can cause Depression—see Part One. Some of these treatments are only short-term (Interferon for a year or so), some are needed for many years (Prednisone), and some can be changed to a different drug (Inderal to another blood pressure pill). High-doses of certain epilepsy medications might make epileptics feel Depressed: Topamax, Dilantin, and Phenobarbital, for example. Certain psychiatric medications can cause Depression in some patients but not in others; for example, major tranquilizers.

Then there are known causes of Depression that are under the patient's control. Street drugs and alcohol can cause Depression. Certain chemicals might cause Depression (glue sniffing and so on). Certain (sedating) herbs (valeriana, kava) might worsen Depression. Some self-destructive compulsive behaviors might cause Depression or may be closely associated: overeating, gambling, and so on.

Some patients decide to stop taking treatments even though they know that stopping the treatment might unleash a Depression. The reasons for stopping treatment can be varied: psychological side effects or intolerance of medication side effects. Some Depressive, schizophrenic, and some neurological patients who already have an underlying Depression may refuse to continue taking a synthetic medication in the belief that the patients can heal the Depression themselves by another method—only to end up more Depressed. They do not care if they make it worse by refusing treatment. This act of not caring is just one more symptom of an underlying Depression. In other cases, non-Depressed patients do not realize that stopping the treatment might result in Depression. Another type of patient finds the treatment to be worse than the disease, and their stated reason for refusing treatment is that they do not care if they become Depressed—that Depression seems better than the original disease and its treatment. This reasoning can occur among end-stage kidney patients who refuse to have dialysis. There are as many reasons for refusing treatments as there are patients.

SECONDARY DEPRESSION DUE TO MEDICAL DISORDER

EIRENE

Eirene was a young woman whose life was going well until she developed a blood disorder requiring the use of moderate dose Prednisone (a prescription steroid). She then became puffy, bloated, apathetic, and Depressed. Her hematologist (blood specialist) sent her to a psychiatrist who prescribed her Lexapro which helped somewhat. Her Depression improved for a while and then deepened, and the doctors all opined that the Prednisone was part of the cause of the Depression. After a few more months, she opted to have surgery (spleen removal) after which her Prednisone was tapered off, but she still felt Depressed. After a few months, lab tests demonstrated that her original condition was only partially better and that she would still need to be on Prednisone—or some other even more toxic drug—for an indefinite period. This was seriously bad news to a young woman who had had many plans for her future life.

She did continue the Prednisone, the dosage of which was lowered slowly over the next few years. Her Depression improved on Lexapro, but she still felt sad, overweight and bloated.

Discussion: This is a case concerning a patient who has no current psychiatric condition, but who does develop a medical condition requiring the use of a medication known to cause mood changes (Prednisone). The blood disorder does not cause Depression, but the drug used to treat it, will cause Depression. There are several such commonly used medical medications with a notorious ability to cause frequent Depressions in medical patients.

The ideal treatment is to remove the cause of the Depression (stop taking Prednisone). But in these cases, that is not possible. Most of these patients have serious medical conditions, which must be treated appropriately. As a result, the Prednisone cannot be stopped, and psychiatrists will need to "treat around" the Prednisone.

Diagnosis: Eirene has a secondary Depression with a known cause, Prednisone.

Treatment: try to control the blood disease, and in the meantime, the Rx is Lexapro. Psychiatrists usually treat these cases "symptomatically"—this means giving medications for whatever symptom that the Prednisone is causing. If Prednisone causes Depression, then an antidepressant is an ideal choice. If the Prednisone is causing mania, then an anti-manic drug is a prime candidate. Likewise, if the Prednisone is causing a psychosis, then an anti-psychotic drug is a good choice. The choice of a specific antidepressant depends on many factors, such as age, gender, other medical problems, other medications, family history (Manic-Depressives in the family), and so on. In Eirene's case, Lexapro is a good choice as it is unlikely to interact with other medications. Any antidepressant or mood stabilizer would be a possible treatment unless that medicine has an undesirable effect on her blood disorder or reacts badly with Prednisone. Wellbutrin also has very little interaction with other medications. There is no FDA-approved antidepressant for Secondary Depression because all the antidepressant medications have been clinically tested only in cases of Primary Depression ("naturally-occurring" Depression). Therefore, the treatment depends exclusively on the psychiatrist's experience and judgment. Patients do not know this fact, which should be explained to them before they become overwrought and waste too many hours doing personal research on the Internet. Cases of Secondary Depression are treated symptomatically.

Outcome: depends upon the severity of the primary medical disorder—if it is severe, she will need higher dose Prednisone, and will have more secondary Depression as well as possible antidepressant side effects due to high dose antidepressant; if the primary medical condition is mild, then she may be able to use only tiny doses of Prednisone, in which case the Lexapro dose might be decreased and any Lexapro side effects should be negligible.

A secondary Depression will usually improve once the cause has been eliminated, after which patients will hopefully go back to their baseline mood (not Depressed). In some cases, the Depression may linger even after the primary disorder is corrected. In Eirene's case, the blood disorder may be permanent, thus the Prednisone will be needed on a long-term basis. If she could be weaned off the Prednisone and not need it anymore, then the Depression might disappear and not come back.

DR. T

Dr. T was a worrywart: he was quite compulsive. He had been a completely normal boy until he had a childhood infection of "Strep throat" resulting in PANDAS (Pediatric Autoimmune Neuropsychiatric Disorder Associated with Streptococcus), after which he seemed to become quite anxious. He was obsessed with symmetry and order. His toy soldiers, Hot Wheels, building blocks, and other toys had to be put into certain arrangements or alignments. This behavior was annoying in his personal life; however, these behaviors propelled him through high school, college, and medical school—and then on into pathology where he was obsessed with pathology slides and collected them in vast numbers. He never took vacations because he was afraid that someone would rearrange his slides, paperwork, and lab in general.

The hospital, St. Elsewhere, unfortunately went "too deep into the red" then went out of business (partly because of huge financial losses from the Emergency Room). Dr. T could not find another job as a pathologist. Worst of all, his supervisor, Dr. A, was offered a transfer to the largest hospital in their group, and A was allowed to take all the hospital property with him (Dr.T's slides). After this, Dr. T stayed at home alone (unmarried, childless) and began to brood. There were no jobs available in pathology at that time. Then he started arranging all the plants in his garden according to his conception of Linnæan botanical classification. He also took his dog on daily hikes in the foothills and canyon.

One morning he awoke with a large round red skin rash which he incredulously recognized as a "target lesion." He went to see Dr. Smith, his family doctor, who confirmed the diagnosis of Lyme Disease and treated T accordingly. With his luck running out, Dr.T developed a complication from the Lyme Disease—it gave him a new kind of anxiety. This second anxiety differed from the one caused by the childhood infection. The Lyme Disease gave him a constant and heightened awareness of his surroundings at all times, resulting in "high anxiety." Eventually, his anxiety resulted in a Depression in which he fretted constantly about everything but accomplished nothing. He could not even do any arranging or aligning or hiking and his house became extremely disorderly. He made frequent visits to Dr. Smith for all types of imagined medical problems that were all a by-product of the intense new high anxiety (see "somatizing" in Vocabulary). Dr. Smith prescribed him Atarax, Benadryl, Valium, Xanax, and Buspar, all to no avail. His doctor insisted that T see a psychiatrist which T resisted doing. As a pathologist who focuses only on diseases that he can examine under a microscope, T thought psychiatry was a "crock." He adamantly refused to see a "quack" or a "shrink."

Then his anxiety became chronic and probably depleted him of his "brain hormones"; then he felt so "burnt out" that he also developed Depressive symptoms, too. His anxious symptoms and Depression continued to fester at home until one day he arose from his over-wrought lethargy and started rearranging the plants, pots, garbage cans, and the garages of his neighbors, which resulted in a longish one-way trip in the back of a police cruiser to the nearest ER (which had not been the nearest ER until St. Elsewhere went bankrupt). T was admitted to the psychiatric ward involuntarily (against his will) and was offered Zyprexa pills which he refused to swallow. He "cheeked" these pills and managed to spit them out on the sly. The medical staff was surprised that he was not improving, and surmised that he was "non-compliant" (not taking his treatment). So, he was changed to Zydis-Zyprexa rapid-dissolving tablets and was reminded that he had a serious mental disorder requiring serious medication; the nurse watched his Zydis dissolve on his tongue. He decided to take this treatment despite a lot of grumbling and renewed protests: he secretly thought, as many patients do, that he would cooperate so as to get out of the hospital as soon as possible, after which he would stop the medication. Luvox was also added. After a week, he actually became much better and was able to go home. Not to say that he was immensely improved, but his outward behavior certainly was, and that is what really counted, as far as the townsfolk and his neighbors were concerned. Contrary to his original plan, he continued taking Luvox and Zyprexa after discharge.

Discussion: yes, infections can cause psychiatric diseases, although this cannot be proven except for the time line. Dr. T has the bad luck to be affected psychiatrically by two serious infections. His first serious infection, strep throat, was a common disease and in this case with an uncommon outcome. "Strep" infections are a rare but possible cause of Obsessive Compulsive Disorder (OCD), an anxiety disorder. Usually OCD has no known cause, except in these cases (childhood "strep" infections).

His second serious infection was Lyme Disease which can cause serious and permanent neuro-psychiatric disorders of any type, prompting doctors to compare it to syphilis, which can similarly cause a multitude of brain aftereffects.

Diagnosis: Secondary Depression (Anxious Depression), probably due to Lyme disease, plus a history of OCD secondary to PANDAS.

Treatment: T went to see his psychiatrist once every month or two for management of Rx medications, Zyprexa and Luvox. Zyprexa is approved for use in Cycling Depressions, but it is also quite useful for anxious Depression and agitated Depression—it is not FDA-approved for these Depressions, but it can be very helpful, anyway. Prescribing Zyprexa for agitated Depression is "off-label" use, which is neither illegal nor unethical, especially since it is a psychiatric medication prescribed by a psychiatrist. Once again, the Secondary Depression is being treated symptomatically, as in the case of Eirene. Luvox is an antidepressant which also has powerful anti-OCD effects. The fact that T needs both of these major medications to remain stabilized is an indicator of the severity of his combined Anxiety and Mood disorders.

Outcome: sometimes when one door closes, another door opens. Dr. T 's compulsive personal quirks that had been annoying behaviors were no longer interfering very much in his personal life. He felt improved enough to call up a nurse whom he had known from his former job. He was able to tolerate the fact that she did not completely understand the precise way in which he ordered his house, but he learned to compromise. He is in his first major relationship, and they are now living together. This may be *As Good as It Gets*, but he may be a lot better off in the long run. (In the movie of the same name, Jack Nicholson had OCD—and narcissism, too, apparently.)

SECONDARY DEPRESSION
DEPRESSION DUE TO ALCOHOL
AND DRUG ADDICTION

Alcohol and street drugs are notorious for causing Depression. Alcohol depresses the brain, so obviously it causes Depression. Furthermore, constant drinking also destroys brain cells. Although we now know that the brain can grow new nerve cells, the brain is hard pressed to try to keep up with the progressive rate of nerve cell destruction caused by serious alcoholism. Anyone with half a brain is not going to feel up to par. Depression is not a surprising outcome of alcoholism. However, alcoholics think that it is. They associate intoxication with feeling "buzzed" and stimulated, and therefore refuse to acknowledge that their alcohol intake causes them any Depression (after the intoxication wears off and they go into alcohol withdrawal).

I occasionally see Depressed alcoholic patients who want me to treat their alcohol-induced Secondary Depression as if it were a naturally occurring Primary Depression. In other words, they will not quit drinking, will not admit that drinking is a problem, and flat-out refuse to consider that alcohol has any relationship to their Depression. They are firmly convinced that their Depression is totally unrelated to alcoholism even though the Depression usually started some time after their drinking went from social drinking to alcoholism.* Their logic here is unclear because this is how alcohol usually causes Depression. But at any rate, they feel perfectly justified in challenging my apparently absurd assumption and illogical diagnostic conclusion regarding the causative role of alcohol in their Depression. They may also turn to a different strategy on the return visit by saying that their drinking started first and that they are "self-treating" Depression with alcohol. This statement, they feel, establishes that they have a Primary Depression, which justifies a trial of an antidepressant. But they still refuse to quit drinking, so where is the cooperation? A third ploy is to toss out the "Bipolar" tactic. This is the commonest contemporary defense to alcoholism and is the modern alcoholic's "default setting," as in "My 'Bipolar' makes me drink." Once again, they are not willing to trade in their alcohol in place of prescription bipolar medication. Regardless of ploy and tactics, they want me to keep on giving them new antidepressants every week or two (while they continue drinking) in order to try to find the one antidepressant that "works" [stops their Depression]—in other words, since the alcohol causes their Depression, they really want me to cure their alcoholism. The first step in treating/curing alcoholic Depression is to treat the underlying primary alcoholism. But, they do not believe themselves to be true alcoholics, so therefore they see no need to quit drinking. And, we reach a philosophical impasse. It is fairly clear from these discussions, that they do not intend to quit drinking while taking an antidepressant—and I usually make it fairly clear that I do not want to prescribe mood-altering medications to practicing alcoholics. Often, they are defensive about their drinking and will not even discuss that at all, in the fear that the psychiatrist will "manipulate" them into "falsely" admitting that alcohol is involved. Some of them even go so far as to assert that alcohol "helps" their Depression. Alcoholism is the only disease that tells its victims that they have no disease—or that it might cure a disease.

What these patients really want is a pill that makes them so euphoric in the daytime that they can stay awake and get a pleasant "buzz" from drinking every evening. The precise outcome of this plan of theirs is that they will be able to continue drinking for another year or two or three while over-stimulated by the antidepressant. As the alcohol makes them more Depressed, they will increase the dose of stimulating antidepressant to offset the effects of the Alcoholic Depression. Eventually, they will be back in my office with the same problem, because the stimulating antidepressant has allowed them to drink ever more, so that now they are even more Depressed every morning and need even higher daily doses of stimulating antidepressant, but then need higher doses of alcohol every night in order to calm down (pass out), and so on: in other words, their alcoholism has worsened and deepened. And their alcoholism will be even harder to treat, not to mention all the physical damage it causes their bodies during that three-year extension of their drinking careers. This merry-go-round will continue until something truly bad happens. This is why I balk at providing aggressive treatment for alcoholic Depression in alcoholics who continue to drink while in treatment.

And so, these patients move on to find another psychiatrist where they craft a better story and omit the part about alcohol. I know this, because some of these patients come to me from their other previous psychiatrists. And some of them do end up receiving Bipolar medications that should not be mixed with alcohol. Eventually, the truth about their drinking habits does surface when they end up drunk in the ER, in court, or when their concerned family members call to express concern about the drinking. Apart from this collateral information, what these patients do not realize is that a lot of psychiatrists have a sixth sense about people's drinking habits based on verbal clues and nonverbal cues.

Street drugs are a separate issue and can cause Depression in many ways. Addiction to stimulants, "uppers," suppresses Depression while the drug is in effect, but when the drug wears off, the original Depression reappears; additionally, a patient, like Rhonda, will have withdrawal from the stimulating drug. The withdrawal appears in the form of a Secondary Depression.

Other people are addicted to sedatives and sleeping pills, "downers." These drugs serve to Depress the brain, with a somewhat similar outcome to that obtained in alcoholism. At least the sedatives do not destroy brain cells as does alcohol. Some people obtain these "downer" drugs illegally, and some, legally on prescription. Occasionally, one of these patients will come from St Elsewhere taking obscene amounts of Valium or Klonopin, and we have a slightly different discussion about weaning off the highly addictive Depressant drug with gradual introduction of an antidepressant (if needed). I usually have the same "philosophical discussions" with drug addicts as with alcoholics. The doctor's advantage in these cases is the power to control access to the addicting drugs by the issuing of prescriptions (whereas the doctor has no control over their access to alcohol). These patients will be advised that they are going to be weaned off the drugs, and each monthly prescription will contain about 10-15% fewer pills or of lower dosage. Patients may do a lot of posturing and acting out, but they know that the pills are addicting and that the dosage is extremely high. They are always free to find another doctor. Apart from being unethical, it is also a violation for California doctors to continue prescribing highly addicting drugs to already-addicted patients—the only quibbling might be over the amount of daily drug that represents an addiction as opposed to routine medical treatment, but we all know about where that boundary lies. (Obscene amounts of Valium are 40 mg a day [for backache or anxiety] and Klonopin 8 mg a day as treatment for anxiety; Klonopin treatment for epilepsy is a separate issue, but if Klonopin were prescribed for epilepsy, then the patient would be seeing a neurologist for the prescription.)

---

*in cases where they report that they were Depressed before drinking started, they might benefit from an antidepressant, but the pill will be useless as long as they continue drinking.

SECONDARY DEPRESSION DUE TO DRUG ADDICTION

RHONDA

Rhonda has a primary problem of drug addiction. She likes any drug or chemical that is mood or mind-altering. When she was in middle school, she started spending her allowance on cough syrup. She liked to drink a whole bottle of cough syrup (containing alcohol) and wait to see if she felt stimulated or sedated—either sensation was fine, as long as she felt altered. She was often sent to see the school nurse. Sometimes she passed out at school. She smoked cigarettes in the girls' bathroom and intimidated any girls who tried to report her. She had formed bonds with a couple other students who were like-minded.

Apart from this, she comes from a stable middle class family. She is an only child, her parents are both successful in their chosen professions, and Rhonda has more freedom than do some students. She also has less parental oversight and feedback.

One of her uncles is an alcoholic who has recovered in A.A. One of her aunts has an on-again/off-again pill addiction and works in the entertainment industry. Her alcoholic grandmother took an accidental overdose of sleeping pills when Rhonda was a girl. One of her distant cousins is in and out of prison (drugs and alcohol are factors in many crimes). There is no history of suicide, overdose, or apparent Depression.

After dropping out of high school, Rhonda moved to Las Vegas and became a "keno" girl. She had an affair with the pit boss who later had her tossed out of the casino. Then she worked "independently" and quickly became a "crystal meth" addict so as to earn as much money as possible. She was thrilled with her "glamorous" life of all-night "partying". However, after two abortions and other medical problems, she came to her senses and determined to lick her addiction. She registered for a six-month stay in a women's sober living home. She soon developed a nagging Depression and felt unmotivated, sad, moody, and empty inside. She was prescribed Remeron at bedtime which helped her sleep well for the first time in years (Remeron is a sedating non-addicting antidepressant). Her Depression quickly resolved and she was able to quit taking it before she left the sober-living home.

Discussion: based on her history, Rhonda comes from a family where addiction is common and Depression is not. Her Depression seemingly follows from the addiction which came first and was her primary problem. After a period of years, the drug addiction depletes her brain of "feel-good" "brain hormones", and this results in a drug-induced Depression. The Depression is secondary to the Addiction, because the Depression began well after the Addiction was already under way.

Diagnosis: amphetamine addiction; Secondary Depression due to amphetamine withdrawal

Treatment: Rhonda quit the antidepressant Remeron after nine months, because she had a relatively mild and brief depressive episode due to stopping a stimulant antidepressant (amphetamine). Depression is not a big issue in her life or in her family history. She continued with her main treatment which was regular attendance at N.A. meetings (Narcotics Anonymous) and affiliated Twelve Steps meetings (Crystal Meth Anonymous).

Outcome: Rhonda felt empowered to go back and finish a two-year program in Cosmetology at the local community college. Rhonda's story shows that one episode of Depression plus drug addiction is not two disabling conditions. She has only one primary diagnosis, amphetamine addiction, which is not a psychiatric disability.

Derek—Drug addiction: see Mixed Depressions / Suicide
Jerrold—Drug addiction: see Mixed Depressions / Suicide
Marc-Evan—Marijuana dependence: see Mixed Depressions

SECONDARY DEPRESSION DUE TO ALCOHOLISM

SASHA (ALEKSANDR):

Minor Depression associated with Alcohol Abuse

Sasha is a Russian émigré who likes his vodka. He has about half a pint of vodka every evening and it makes him feel warm inside and content. He is not an alcoholic but is at times a heavy drinker. He does not feel morning remorse or have blackouts like a true alcoholic. He does not pass out at night and "come to" in the morning like a real alcoholic. He is, however, prone to irritable outbursts whether drinking or not. His liver function is not [yet] significantly altered, his bone marrow is unaffected, and he has gained little weight partly because he is quite active, playing soccer on the weekends. Yet already his cholesterol levels are mildly elevated and his skin looks puffy and sallow. After many years of vodka drinking, he has recently begun to notice that he feels depressed the next morning.

He consults his family doctor every couple months about minor aches and pains, tiredness on Monday mornings, strange dreams, and decreased interest in sex (see "somatizing" in the Vocabulary). His doctor, who is not fully aware of all the vodka intake, finally gives Sasha some Zoloft which seems to start helping him within a couple weeks. After a couple months, Sasha feels better with Zoloft. He is more active and pleasant and has more interest in activities. He has better focus and concentration. After a few months, his wife remarks that overall he seems to be coming "into focus"; he looks better and seems less "puffy." After several months, he begins to note that he is not drinking very much at all on the weekday evenings, has a couple vodka cocktails on Saturday evening, and maybe a beer or two on Sunday afternoons.

Discussion of possible diagnoses: Sasha has a mild Depression and daily alcohol consumption. What is the association? Did alcohol cause the Depression or did the Depression cause alcohol abuse? Or are they separate conditions? He drank for years before feeling Depressed, thus his Depression appeared later and could be caused by alcohol because of the timeline. After he began to feel Depressed, he may have tried to treat himself by ramping up the daily drinking; the fact that evening cocktails make him feel stimulated and chatty may have further reinforced this impression. At any rate, he starts Zoloft and his Depressive symptoms do clear up (along with simultaneous reduction in alcohol consumption). If Sasha quits drinking altogether and then later quits taking Zoloft and remains non-Depressed, then we can assume that he had a Secondary Depression due to alcohol abuse (a temporary Depression) because both conditions disappeared. Another possibility is that he quits drinking but the Depression continues. What is the source of this residual Depression? It could have been caused by alcohol abuse but now persists as a permanent Minor Depression; or, the Depression could have arisen "naturally" as a primary Depression and has nothing to do with alcohol. However, we know that alcohol can cause Depression or worsen a Depression. In this case, he needs treatment for both conditions—he needs to quit drinking (treatment for alcohol abuse) and to continue Zoloft (treatment for Depression). He might also benefit from some therapy sessions or a dozen AA meetings, but most of these men like Sasha will balk at such treatment suggestions.

In real-life practice, few patients quit drinking totally; most of these patients cut down on their drinking, continue the Zoloft, and feel better. They report that attempts to quit drinking make them feel Depressed; likewise, they report that quitting Zoloft makes them Depressed.

Diagnostic possibilities as listed above: (1) Secondary Depression due to temporary alcohol abuse; (2) chronic Depression with ongoing alcohol abuse as a self-treatment; or, (3) Sasha has two primary disorders of mild Major Depression and of alcohol abuse, that are two separate diagnoses.

Treatment: the ideal treatment in all three diagnostic possibilities is to quit alcohol completely and take antidepressants if and only if Depression persists.

Outcome: good-very good in case (1); fair in case (2); fair to poor, regardless of exact diagnosis, in case (3); most of these patients completely overlook the vodka as a possible cause of Depression since it makes them feel jolly every evening. They miss the connection, because the morning depression is half a day removed from cocktail hour. Their spouses, however, sometimes aptly make the connection.

SECONDARY DEPRESSION DUE TO ALCOHOLISM

ALBERTO

Alberto works as kitchen staff in a Mexican restaurant in East Los Angeles where he is used and abused by the management. He is paid less than a living wage and works overtime without overtime pay. He is an illegal alien from Central America and feels very isolated despite living with five other bachelors in a small house near the restaurant. Two of the others are from his homeland, one of whom grew up with Alberto in the same village.

He is a survivor of political upheaval in his small country. During the last revolution, Alberto lost his father, uncle, and elder brothers one by one, to various causes. Alberto grew up with his mother, sisters, and grandfather who were not members of the privileged class. Their tiny farm was illegally seized by a local landlord, and they all ended up moving to the capital and living in a *casa de cartón* (makeshift lean-to in a seriously poor slum).

When Alberto reached teenage years, he had no prospects for employment or future life. He and his mother went to the American embassy to apply for political asylum based on their family situation, but the paperwork disappeared into an abyss. So, he—like other young men—resolved to go to California to seek a better life where he found a typical arrangement of young bachelors who were living together in very cramped quarters and sharing space—up to four per bedroom. They were all working illegally to make a small amount of money that they would wire back to their families in their countries of origin. This was basically his life in L.A.

Once every weekend, Alberto and a couple companions would buy some beer and drink up a small part of their earnings, finding hours of fellowship cushioned in the warmth of familiarity. A pleasant experience of "social lubrication" provided by the liquid drug, alcohol, helped soothe his sadness at being in a new land so far away from home. And then he started to binge on the weekends and forgot to send money back to his mother. It is not certain when Alberto became alcoholic, but it seemed to be rather quickly. Although Alberto started spiraling down into early alcoholism, he was still able to hold down his job and work long hours. By way of sheer luck, one of the waiters in the restaurant, Beto, was a recovering alcoholic who noted Alberto's drinking problem and strongly suggested that Alberto accompany him to a *junta de "doble-A"* (AA meeting), in order to avoid losing his job. Alberto grudgingly agreed, partly because he had much to lose by continued drinking. Actually, AA became Alberto's major social outing and was a real bargain, costing him a dollar or less per meeting. Attending this one meeting had no effect on Alberto's drinking, but he noted that there were some attractive young women in the meeting, and this observation piqued his interest such that he was looking forward to returning to the same meeting one week later. Eventually, he was able to quit drinking altogether, one week at a time. His life got better in AA because next he met Maria at a meeting and they eventually were married.

Unfortunately, he started to become Depressed during the first year of sobriety. The Depression worsened and then Alberto was in danger of losing his job due to the Depression. He consulted a doctor from his homeland and was started on Ludiomil, which helped him to feel complete and competent again. He took it for a couple years and had tried to quit taking it on a few occasions, but always slipped back into an irritable Depression, whereupon Maria would insist that he resume the medication. The bad news was that a permanent psychiatric condition seemingly had occurred in his brain. The good news was that Ludiomil made him feel 85% better. He had acquired a permanent persistent but manageable Depression. He continued to go to an AA meeting every week or two.

Discussion: He began first with a minor and temporary Reactive Depression, which he started to treat with alcohol. This gave him a minor and temporary diagnosis of "Alcohol abuse," which does not cause permanent changes in the brain. If Alcohol Abuse is not corrected, however, it can progress into full-blown Alcoholism which becomes a permanent brain disease, which in this case was followed by a permanent Depression (chronic Major Depression). Whether his untreated Reactive Depression became a Secondary Depression, or whether the Depression arose independently, he still ended up with a chronic Major Depression.

Sometimes such a Major Depression will disappear in sobriety (as in Rhonda's case), and sometimes, it will not (Alberto).

Lack of access to health care increases the risk of the worsening of a disease such as Depression. Having multiple psychological and social stress factors can also evolve into a Major Depression. In his case, these stresses are political upheaval, socio-economic instability, multiple family deaths, emigration to a foreign country, and a low-level service sector job. (Alcoholism is sometimes considered to be a "spiritual" disease as well as an emotional and physical brain disease.)

Diagnosis: Alcoholism and Mild Major Depression; multiple grief reactions for multiple losses of father, brothers, and homeland.

Treatment: continue Ludiomil and AA meetings

Outcome: is good as long as he follows treatment guidelines; his outcome is poor if he does not continue to take care of his mental health by maintaining his spiritual and emotional balance. If he quits the antidepressant, he might sink further into Depression at which point he might resume drinking alcoholically. If an alcoholic resumes drinking, he is not capable of drinking socially and will most likely drink to excess every night. On the other hand, if Alberto continues the Ludiomil but drops out of AA, then he may likely go into a "dry drunk" stage in which he will show evidence of many of his drinking behaviors: he will become irritable, resentful, suspicious, and fly off the handle frequently. He may be tense and likely to flare up over any minor annoyance that would not affect him if he were sober. He will also obsess and worry about everything.

Gilbert—Alcoholism: read his story under Major Depression ("Dual Diagnosis")
Dolores—read about her use of alcohol under Major Depression, "Chronic Depression"

DEPRESSIONS
ASSOCIATED WITH CHILD ABUSE

This topic is best discussed as not one Depression, but rather as "Depressions." Most adults who have suffered child abuse will have more than one Depression or they may have one type of Depression plus PTSD with/without alcoholism/drug-abuse. PTSD is an anxiety disorder than occurs in people who have been exposed to extraordinary stress factors in their lives (child sex abuse, in this case). When these children grow up, they commonly turn to alcohol and drugs to suppress bad memories; this form of self-treatment backfires for women as it may decrease their judgment about their dealings with men; this form of self-treatment backfires in men if it results in violent sprees in which they act out their rage. Not all sexually abused children grown up to have alcohol and drug problems, but many of them have family history of alcoholism and drug addiction.

TIFFANY

Her mother abandoned the family very early in Tiffany's life, and Tiffany brought herself up. She lived in the same house with her father, uncle, and elder half-brother, but they did not rear her—no one did, in fact. At a very early age she had been abused almost nightly by one or all of these male relatives, all of whom fit somewhere into the rubric of alcoholism. Her mother's twin sister, Tammie-Lea had tried for years to get custody of Tiffany and finally ended up paying Tiffany's father to sign over custody—and he agreed.

After barely graduating high school, Tiffany decided to take off for Hollywood and try her hand at making money there. She ended up in the San Fernando Valley, the Hollywood of the Pornography Industry.

She worked there for over a year in various positions, but was merely going through the motions; the pay was very good and she was saving as much money as she could.

One day she stopped into a nice up-scale diner to have a calorie-controlled snack. Tiffany saw a nice young couple in the restaurant—a young woman similar to herself but who had nice clothes, a polished and poised demeanor, and—most importantly—a handsome young man who was very communicative and attentive. They left the restaurant in a BMW convertible. Then Tiffany decided that she would forget her diet and get a tuna melt and coconut cream pie. Tiffany thought nothing more of this and went home to take a "disco nap" alone in her hardscrabble studio apartment in a seamier neighborhood of Van Nuys.

She slept much longer than expected and awoke at midnight awash in horrible new feelings of emptiness like a spiritual vacuum. She suddenly realized that she would probably never earn a college degree from USC or UCLA, or have a good job, and would likely never have a nice life and a handsome boyfriend with a BMW convertible. She was so overwhelmed with this emotional tsunami that she felt paralyzed and lay on her futon as if her whole body were flattened against it. She had no force to get up or even to move in the slightest degree. Disgusting memories of her worst moments in life repeatedly savaged her soul and thus she lay for the whole night, seemingly. She wasn't sure if she had *never* felt this way before or if she had never *allowed* herself to feel this way before. At any rate, this debate inside her head did nothing to change the fact that she was awash in ill feelings and undertowed by the sudden overwhelming flood of empty Depression.

She still felt drenched in Depression the next morning and dreaded the thought of going to work at the film studio. After one difficult and especially trying day, she stopped on her way home to buy a bottle of Benadryl at the all-night pharmacy. As if in a trance, she took the bottle of pills home and—without forethought—she knew what she must do: take the whole bottle of pills so as to sleep well—and perhaps sleep forever. She had no definite plans…just to escape for a while…or for a little while longer than that, …or for however long that might be… that she might need that respite—she didn't care at that point.

The next afternoon, she came to, in a very groggy state and then went back to sleep or passed out again, depending upon one's viewpoint of the whole episode. She knew what she must do next: go back to live with her aunt Tammie-Lea and try to sort out her life. Shortly after arriving there, she took another excessive dose of Benadryl. Her aunt called the EMS, and Tiffany woke up next in the hospital where she stayed overnight. It was decided that she would be set up for an urgent intake evaluation at the county mental health clinic.

Tiffany thus began a long and difficult journey to try to connect her past with her present and future. She was assigned an older female therapist whom she saw regularly for years to come. She spent the next few years trying to steer clear of the world of men. Her dating prospects were marginal at best, since she was hounded by her past and handicapped by her present confusion. And, although she had a few romantic disappointments, the worst disappointments were those fantasy dates that never even eventuated in a first date, nor in association with the previously mentioned German convertible.

She was stabilized on Celexa and Trazodone and even started attending Alanon meetings, which were also very helpful. She even got her first boyfriend, who was a few years younger—and he even had a convertible. It was a Mustang. It felt good to ride around Centerville while supporting Detroit.

Discussion: These are complicated cases of people who require many years or decades to recover. More than one form of Depression may be present, and there is almost always more than one psychiatric diagnosis present. One problem is that of a lost childhood. Another problem is that of the sexual abuse. A lost childhood cannot be replaced.

Diagnosis: Depression and PTSD.

Treatment: supportive talk therapy, occupational rehabilitation and continue Celexa and Trazodone

Outcome: good in general but only fair in regards to long-term relationships; she is not disabled. Tiffany continued in treatment for years and made huge strides and progress. She became a hairdresser, eventually moving in with her Mustang lover, and later they eased into a self-declared common-law marriage.

MARC-EVAN

Marc was the middle child of three, between elder brother Tim and sister Aimée. Marc always felt that he lived in Tim's shadow, or at least as far as his parents were concerned. Tim excelled at athletics and scholastics and was quite popular in school. Marc's boyhood was defined by lackluster participation in Little League. He had dropped out of Boy Scouts after attaining first class [rank] and a few merit badges. His endeavors were characterized by loss of interest and lack of follow-through. He had trouble finishing anything that he started and often felt confused, isolated, withdrawn, unmotivated, and sad despite being with people. A number of his crayoned pictures were traced in gray tones with only one spot of red or yellow.

Both his parents drank socially, entertained a lot, and often traveled for business, leaving Marc and Tim in the care of their older cousin, Micah, who lived two blocks away. Micah was involved in basketball and somewhat popular, but also slightly "different"—which Marc's parents referred to as being "artistic." Micah had girlfriends but was also bisexual, and liked to bully Marc. Micah started sexually abusing Marc when Marc was quite young and this continued off and on until Micah graduated from high school and went off to college.

Marc likewise had artistic tendencies and even went so far as to join Art Club, but tended to be a loner. Marc empathized with the "loadies" and Goths, but also gravitated toward the "cycle bums," as Marc's father called them. Marc did not feel that he really fit in with any certain club or group, and was, in principal, a loner. He had one best friend, Raj, who lived next door and with whom he shared such common interests as archery, golf, science projects, and backyard rocketry. Raj attended summer school each year and graduated when he was sixteen years old. He went off to college, and Marc felt lonely again.

By the end of high school, Marc's tastes changed slowly as he gravitated toward a much more "Bohemian" crowd. He was smoking marijuana almost daily. He began to see his parents as ridiculously "bourgeois" and secretly began referring to his mother as "Mrs. Robinson" when she started having poolside martinis and wearing a bikini to swim with Tim's friends.

Around this time, Micah moved back to LA to attend graduate school and moved back in with his parents temporarily. Micah came over one evening with beer and marijuana when Marc's parents were gone for the weekend. Micah and Marc were apparently drinking heavily and Marc blacked out. The next morning, he and Micah woke up naked in bed together, each with a couple bruises. Marc deduced that Micah and he at some point had been swigging Nyquil and bourbon, based on the trail of empty bottles leading into the bathroom. The rest of the night was essentially forgotten, but Marc began to suspect what might have gone down—and, also that Micah had not "reformed" despite being engaged.

Hung over and very confused, Marc managed to kick Micah out of the house and then sought solace by picking the lock on his parents' liquor closet. He had decided that he did not want to think about anything or try to remember anything at that moment on that day, as many dark memories came back to haunt his waking hours. Mark spent the rest of the day drinking more liquor and stayed in bed for twenty hours. 'My life is ruined...' this one thought haunted him obsessively day and night. He could not even select an emotion to have, but he was afraid that a homicidal rage might emerge, so he stayed drunk for as long as he could.

Soon thereafter, Marc struck up a relationship with twenty-two-year old Dianna who complained that Marc always had to be stoned to have sex with her. The relationship had its up's and down's and really did not take off, despite many months living together on the weekends. "It bothers me that you can only have sex with me if you smoke first? Why is that?!" she quizzed him. He reacted with a sudden outpouring of rage. He sought a hard target and punched a hole in the wall. After a few moments of silent reflection, she mumbled, "I hope you didn't give me AIDS!" Then she moaned dismally at this sudden realization, anticipating this possibly unavoidable outcome of their "situationship." Marc was feeling so enraged by this by this remark that belittled him —and so psychotic that he did not feel any pain—that he had to leave the room and went racing out: he knew that he would be awash in great crimson folds of pain and remorse and sought to drench that pain, and so he slammed down great glurgs of hard liquor, drinking straight out of the bottle until he felt hammered, whereupon he went back into the bedroom, throwing himself on the bed. "No, I'm not gay and yes, I like having sex on grass—and that's all..." he softly and slowly slurred and then passed out merely to awaken alone hours later in a cold dark room, emotionally splayed in the penumbra of his rapidly fleeting youth. After that incident, Dianna left the relationship and Marc sank into a deep melancholy which he treated frequently with alcohol and marijuana. He continued to muddle along, often feeling aimless.

After that relationship was over, he would spend a long time staring into the mirror repeatedly trying to analyze the reflection for telltale signs of a repulsive moral malignancy. He tried to see if Micah's abuse had left some telltale signs on his face or body that would be apparent to everyone. Even when he felt certain that there were no such signs, he still growled out, 'It's all Micah's fault!' almost gloatingly blaming Micah, as if Marc had sleuthed around and uncovered a simple explanation to this consumptive and complex secret. And then he sighed, "Yeah, keep telling yourself that."

After that he began to realize that he was or had become gay, he was unsure of which. He toned down the drinking and drugging on his own. During this time, he limited himself to "emergency sex" with other men—brief, anonymous, and infrequent. He had enrolled in community college and had a minor outburst on campus. It scared him enough to seek counseling voluntarily, and his main topic of concern was whether Micah had made him gay, or if it had occurred spontaneously without any known cause. And also, how to continue having sex with women, a "state of success" that Micah had apparently achieved.

After more college studies, Marc was finally accepted into a Master's degree program and after finishing that, he allowed himself to relax and eventually fall in love with Dave, who was destined to become Marc's long-term live-in lover. Marc had finally come to accept himself as he was—this was his life-saving act of humility.

Discussion: Marc was apparently born with Dysthymia, a depressive personality style of people who seem timid and withdrawn with poor self-esteem. By high school, Marc began to evidence new symptoms suggestive of adolescent Depression, such as sullenness, low frustration tolerance, irritability, antisocial outbursts, and—of course—self-treating with chemicals or other compulsive behaviors. Marc's moodiness is no exception. This he unsuccessfully self-treats with marijuana.

He develops a serious marijuana habit that makes him worse. He must quit the marijuana, his drug of choice, which he loves so much. He has grief over the loss of the drug and its effects.

Sexual abuse by an older male does not cause homosexuality. If Marc turned out gay, it is because he was born that way, evidence that he—like Micah—was "artistic." They may share some genetics in this regard. Heterosexual boys who are homosexually abused still grow up to be heterosexual—but most of them are extremely angry and often become heavy abusers of drugs and alcohol in their attempts to erase those past memories that are like waking nightmares that haunt them constantly and drive them to compulsive self-destructive behaviors— all of which furthers the cycles of self-loathing. Apart from all this, slavishly trying to classify human sexuality in strict and rigid terms is practically useless as sexuality is very complex and often hard to classify. The Kinsey Report gave us our first inklings of that and much more research has been done since then.

Diagnosis: Marc has Dysthymia and compulsive marijuana abuse. He also has repressed anger about the sexual abuse.

Treatment: Marc engaged in individual psychotherapy with a therapist until he was able to sort out some of his anger; he also attended treatment for marijuana abuse/addiction and benefited from Effexor-XR and a gay men's therapy group.

Outcome: is good as long as he follows through with these treatments; if he falters, then he may easily relapse, and then his outcome would be only poor-fair. He has one addiction already, so he can easily become cross-addicted to alcohol, cocaine, and other medications: this could lower his outcome to poor.

JERROLD

He grew up in a somewhat dysfunctional and financially strapped family. He had always been very bookish and slight of stature and spent all of his time excelling at natural sciences. In other words, he had no playmates and did not play sports. His family was also "eccentric," to say the least. He had a girlfriend and there was some suspicion that he had slapped her around on more than one occasion.

Jerrold had been sexually abused by his uncle Beau from ages six to twelve. Both of Jerrold's parents had to work long hours, so Uncle

Beau, who was on permanent disability for back pain, became Jerrold's babysitter. Beau had told him one set of lies after another until Jerrold finally figured out that Beau was bad for him. Jerrold became an excellent science student in his high school as a result of which he was awarded a scholarship to Great State University. At the end of his junior year, he began to dabble in marijuana; that did not appear to affect his grades, although it made his behaviors strange (or stranger). During his senior year, he had to work part-time, so he found a job in a pharmacy where he had access to several antidepressants, including Parnate, Marplan, Eutonyl, and Nardil (potent antidepressants); he started taking them without a prescription. Since he had no legal prescription, he would take one of them for a month or two and if supplies were low, then he would switch to another one.

He took a sudden turn for the worse in his senior year of high school and unexpectedly enrolled at the local community college instead of attending Great State University. This was partly so that he could get an apartment and live together with his girlfriend, Marjo, who was in her junior year of high school. (Perhaps it was also to maintain his supply of antidepressants and marijuana.) However, a couple months later, Marjo turned up in the local ER with a black eye and bruises, after which she stayed with her parents. On the day when she and her brother came to the apartment to move her stuff out, they found Jerrold dead on the couch surrounded by empty pill bottles. Everyone was baffled by this turn of events. The coroner's inquest turned up no other information.

Discussion: Jerrold had problems: childhood sexual abuse, drug abuse, and an apparent—but undiagnosed—primary psychiatric problem (most likely Depression). As far as childhood homosexual abuse, heterosexual men can be seriously damaged psychologically by these memories, resulting in anger, violence, Depression, PTSD symptoms (Post-Traumatic Stress Disorder), and alcohol-drug abuse. They can exhibit violence toward self (impulsive acting-out, extremely poor self-care) or toward others (date rape, physical abuse, repeated bar-brawling, homicide).

As far as drug abuse, marijuana can cause Depression, agitation, and confusion. Typical to these cases, Jerrold was probably attempting to suppress bad childhood memories of sexual abuse. Marijuana might also have served as an aphrodisiac, but this is doubtful, since few teenage boys ever need aphrodisiacs (unless antidepressants cause partial impotence).

As far as psychiatric problems, we may assume that Jerrold was Depressed because he was taking antidepressants on the sly. Presumably, he thought he was Depressed. Perhaps he knew the reason for his Depression (sexual abuse?) or maybe he felt great emotional turmoil without being aware of any cause. Two-thirds of suicides are due to Depression; other psychiatric causes of suicide at this age may be schizophrenia or Manic Depression. Schizophrenia and Manic Depression can start at this age in young men; antidepressants and street drugs could have aggravated a manic or psychotic state and caused him to feel suicidal. However, there was no clear-cut evidence that he was developing such serious psychiatric illnesses (as in the movie *Beautiful Mind*), unless he was already "quietly psychotic" or unless he had suddenly become extremely psychotic (called "fulminant" cases). None of that appeared to be the case here.

There are also other infrequent causes of suicide: young men have been known to make suicidal gestures after a romantic disappointment, especially in cases of all-consuming obsessive love: he must have loved Marjo intensely, because he seemingly gave up his scholarship in order to be with her. (Also see topic of Black Box warnings.)

Diagnosis: The diagnosis is unknown but is probably Depression, probably related to PTSD and childhood (homo)sexual abuse. Drug abuse is a contributing factor. He was abusing not only marijuana but also prescription drugs, as demonstrated by his taking antidepressants randomly and without medical oversight.

Treatment: Self-treatment (with chemicals) is the most frequent choice of these men because the vile and tormenting memories must never be discussed—with anyone. This, of course, leads to more of the same and worsening of symptoms. The usual and usually recommended professional treatments for these cases are for anger management, drug treatment, and medication evaluation. Anger management groups should be a rigorous and regular part of the treatment for men with these problems. Specialized men's groups are sometimes available in larger cities. Drug treatment programs would have helped him get off marijuana. As far as medications, there is no one specific FDA-approved treatment for cases like this. We use symptomatic treatment: Depakote,

Zyprexa, or Seroquel for anger; non-stimulating antidepressants for depressive symptoms; and, Buspar or Vistaril for anxiety.

Outcome: these tragedies must be prevented through better mental health education, and early recognition of child abuse. The only currently known effective treatment for compulsive sexual abusers (like Uncle Beau) is the legal remedy of removing the perpetrator from general society by incarceration. This case shows how great plans and great promise can be derailed by great psychological trauma. We can speculate that, but for Uncle Beau, Jerrold might have gone on to be an excellent scientist.

MIXED DEPRESSIONS

These are cases of people who have more than one type of psychiatric diagnosis or more than one type of Depression, but do not have the special combinations called Dual Diagnosis Depression (see Alberto and Gilbert) or Double Depression (see Gilbert and Geb).

AIMÉE

Aimée is the younger sister of Marc-Evan and Tim. She grew up admiring both her brothers. She had always quietly empathized with Marc's "dark" side and silently admired Tim's "bright side." She also knew that both of them had very different weaknesses. She seemed to be the only person who saw them as they really were. As she approached maturity, she had a brief bout with alcoholism around the end of college and in her early twenties. During this whirlwind, she met Harley who seemed to have the stability of her father, the popularity of Tim, and the sensitivity of Marc. Which was to say that Harley had his contemplative and pensive side as well as his bright and gregarious side. She married Harley and had a daughter. During this time, she switched slowly from alcohol to religion while he was furthering his career.

As time went on, she became more obsessed with religion and astrology whereas Harley started to show obvious mood cycles suggestive of Manic-Depression. During his "happy moods," he would be very productive and was involved in all sorts of business deals and schemes. During his "resting moods," he would stay home in bed and avoid social engagements, neglect business opportunities, forget appointments, delay phone calls, and shun social activities in general. Aimée's devotion to religion and the occult and Harley's refusal to seek help for his obvious psychiatric problem created a rift that resulted in divorce. She remarried much later, while he continued to cycle for the next twenty years until his business schemes resulted in court-ordered psychiatric treatment.

Later in life, she reflected back on some of her choices and realized that alcohol abuse might have blurred her judgment. She blamed alcohol indirectly and herself directly for allowing this to happen—especially when she saw her friends marry successful men and have comfortable lives. This sense of regret led her into a state of feeling tired and she felt that her life was a transition that she had endured within the four walls of her small home. Her brother Marc repeatedly urged her to see a doctor about these feelings. She finally did see her family doctor who prescribed her Celexa. She started to feel calm, focused, and motivated. She met a man at church and after three years of dating, they were married there. She became less obsessive about religion and learned to find balance in her life. But she always looked forward to buying a new outfit for Easter each year.

Discussion: Although Aimée has only minor Depression, she comes from a family with Depression. This can affect her choice of friends and boyfriends. Growing up with her brothers may have a part in causing her to gravitate toward Harley. She is compulsive about religion whereas her brother Tim has his own compulsions. This compulsiveness is probably on a genetic basis and not due to pure chance. Aimée comes from a family that suffers Depression as well as Depression-equivalent disorders (alcohol abuse and other compulsions)

Diagnosis: compulsive traits initially manifested as compulsive alcohol abuse, which were then channeled into low-grade religious fanaticism; Minor Depression becomes a mild Major Depression; there is a family history of Depressive and compulsive "temperaments."

Treatment: continue Celexa; she should not drink because her alcohol abuse, which is lying dormant, could progress into alcoholism if she starts drinking heavily. Her brother Marc attends Twelve Steps programs for marijuana dependence, and her brother, Tim, is in and out of GA and SLAA. No further treatment is necessary unless she feels worse or her behaviors interfere significantly with her functioning in general.

Outcome: very good; however, she outlived her second husband, and her daughter forced her into a nursing home at age eighty-six because of early dementia with Depression; Aimée continued low doses of Celexa along with Alzheimer's medicines. Her family history and personal history place her at higher risk of developing some type of Depression in later life, Alzheimer's with Depression, in this case.

MEG

Meg's father died when she was six years old. She and her mother then moved in with two spinster aunts. By the time that Meg was ten, she had changed and was not quite the happy carefree child that she had been. Her school grades remained quite good because she really enjoyed her lessons, although she distanced herself from her teachers and held herself apart from most of the other students. As more time went by, Meg became shier and more socially withdrawn, but functioned well at home, becoming very close to her great-aunts.

Meg's mother found a good job rather far away, so her mother stayed in the city during the week. Meg's mother tried to come home every weekend. Meg's mother's best friend was Dottie, and when Dottie later got a good job in Los Angeles, Meg's mother wanted to move there, too, and made plans to relocate Meg, but Meg's aunts objected, as they felt that Meg was rather "emotionally fragile." This debate went on for months, with the result that Meg would stay with her great-aunts to finish out the school year.

Around this time, Meg became very withdrawn and brooding. She stayed in her room more and played less. She seemed sadder. The school nurse referred her for counseling, and with time, Meg slowly returned to her baseline. Everyone agreed that Meg should stay with her aunts until she graduated high school. She was not started on an antidepressant until she decided to give consent for it. She took it and started to improve.

Meg graduated high school and enrolled in a small local college and continued to live with the aunts. She felt comfortable on a small campus in a small town, and about one third of the college students were already known to Meg from high school. She also made some new acquaintances. She felt grounded as long as she was taking her medication. She started spending a few weeks a year with her mother and Dottie in L.A. She always felt overwhelmed with L.A. and was always glad to return to her life in a small town. Soon, she met a young man, Yves, and they decided to get married and live in the city.

She had four sons who were normal rowdy boys and they interacted a lot with their father, but she never really was able to understand them very well. After the second son was born, she had "baby blues," which recurred with the third son also. After the fourth son, she had a serious Post-partum Depression that required two weeks of psychiatric hospitalization and her mother-in-law drove down from Québec to stay with them for a few months. After the post-partum Depression, Meg started to have Depressions every year, starting in November and lasting until spring. Her psychiatrist treated her with Vital-Lites™ Photo-therapy (artificial sunlight) which was quite effective for her. As the years went by, the Depression seemed to linger all year long but worsened every winter. Therefore, she was taking Wellbutrin all year long plus phototherapy in the winter. Overall, she continued about the same, but was prone to an additional grief Depression after Yves died.

Discussion and Diagnosis: Meg developed a dysthymia after her father died. Then she had a Reactive Depression when her mother moved to California with Dottie. Meg had effectively lost both her parents. This left her more vulnerable to Depression later in life. In her case, she also suffered post-partum Depression and also developed Winter Depression that evolved into a Major Depression. Additionally, she never learned to relate to sons, possibly from losing her father and being brought up by aunts. Childhood Dysthymia can set up some people to have a Depressive reaction to major stressors in later life.

Treatment: continue photo-therapy and medications

Outcome: fair; anyone with these many Depressions will never fully recover and return to baseline personality, but at least with modern treatments, a state of relative comfort can be achieved.

SUICIDE

"**Suicide**" means killing oneself. A committed suicide has already happened and the person has died from the suicide attempt. Suicide is an unfortunate but possible outcome of any major form of Depression. Most Depressions do not end in suicide, but most suicides are the end-stage of one of the major Depressions. A minority of suicides are the result of duress (at gunpoint), self-sacrifice, carelessness-recklessness, "diminished capacity" (intoxication), or deliberate avoidance of extreme and horrible consequences, such as life imprisonment, etc. In one sense, suicide is a case of Terminal Depression.

If we take suicide at its literal meaning of "self-killing" (in Latin), then we can further classify suicides based on the presence or absence of intention.

- Actively Intentional due to Depression: this accounts for an estimated two-thirds of all suicides (this is what we all classically think of when we think of suicide)
- Passively Intentional (cancer patient's refusal to continue chemotherapy, a kidney patient's refusal to continue dialysis, an AIDS patient who makes a conscious decision to quit taking all HIV medications and treatments)
- Preemptively Intentional: self-sacrifice so that others may live
- Unintentional due to mental illness (Schizophrenia): the voices tell a person that he is now Superman and that he is capable of flying off of tall buildings
- Unintentional due to poor judgment (diminished capacity while very intoxicated): repeatedly jaywalking or driving while drunk

- Unintentional while neither intoxicated nor mentally ill: voluntarily engaging in very dangerous activities that "normal" people know to be possibly-probably lethal, such as hang-gliding, asphyxiation-orgasm, freewheeling down steep mountain roads, playing "chicken" with trains, and so on
- Non-intentional: making a dramatic statement that is intended to be a manipulative and non-lethal gesture but results in death anyway: making a suicide gesture after being jilted (Matt); or, Depressives who want to sleep continuously for the whole weekend and then wake up Monday morning feeling "refreshed" (Tiffany);
- Voluntary Political statement (Irish hunger-strikers, Vietnamese Buddhist monks setting themselves on fire[self-immolation])
- Involuntary under duress: in ancient Rome when the praetorian guard was en route to your villa, in ancient China when the emperor sent a silk cord, hari-kari in Japan, threats from mobsters ("shoot yourself or we will all rape you, then slowly stab you")

In this topic, we are discussing only psychiatric suicide. Suicide is among the commonest causes of death in certain age groups (teenage boys and young men). Some suicides are preventable and some are not. A person, who really wants to kill himself, simply does so; if no one knows of his plan, then no one can prevent it. In some cases, the risk of suicide can be decreased by certain interventions.

The underlying foundations for suicide start with having a persistent psychiatric or medical condition. Most persistent psychiatric conditions can result in Depression due to brain 'burn-out" associated with major and chronic Depressions. If the person also has a chronic medical condition or dangerous compulsive disorder, in addition to the Depression, then this merely worsens the odds for a terminal outcome. Since the brain is a physical organ, any medical disease that affects the physical body could affect the physical organ of the brain itself. Good examples of such chronic medical conditions are: multiple sclerosis, HIV-AIDS, chronic pain, cancer, and so on. In one sense, chronic conditions are not really the first stage toward suicide since most people with Depression, cancer, or AIDS neither want to kill themselves, nor want to die; but, in another sense, they may already be in the first stage of suicide because a significant fraction of these people develop a Secondary Depression, and any type of Depression can raise the risk of suicide. Furthermore, Depressives usually have multiple major problems besides just Depression.

There are various steps leading up to suicide. The first step is "passive death wish" followed by the next steps: suicidal ideation, suicidal intention, suicide gesture, suicide attempt, and finally committed suicide. Passive death wish is a symptom of hopelessness expressed when a person makes statements such as: "I wish I were dead," "I would be better off if I were dead," "Oh, why was I ever born?!", "Today might be a good day to die, but I don't really want to kill myself," "I have been such a burden to friends and family," and so on. Passive death wish means that a person is questioning the value of his life, but has no specific plans to do anything at all.

The second step is suicidal ideation, which means researching possible methods that could be used. Women usually prefer a non-violent method, such as overdosing, and may start to accumulate pills. Men prefer methods that are more violent (hence usually lethal): guns, hanging, and accidents. A middle-aged Depressive who suddenly decides to buy his first gun may be in trouble from untreated emotional turmoil.

Third step is intention, which means that the person is making plans. If her plan is overdose, she has the intention to go on-line to read about overdosing: which pills are dangerous, how many are required, and so on. If she buys pills on-line and has the pills sent to her, then she is seemingly serious about going on to the fourth step, which is gesture. She might make a gesture by taking a dose that is not quite lethal but will result in her sleeping for a couple days, thereby allowing her tired Depressed brain to rest: this may have been her real goal, not suicide. If she takes the pills at her parents' house on a Sunday morning, knowing that her family will come home from church and find her passed out, then this is not a true desire to die because she knows that they will find her and call an ambulance—she is counting on their arrival home. One way that this type of gesture can be unintentionally fatal is in the unexpected situation where none of the family comes home until late that night. Many of the people who gesture with pills are really trying to turn off their brains. Other "gesturers" are crying out for help: "Help me! Something is wrong with me! Something is wrong in my life!" A gesture is not intended to be lethal, but most gesturers know that it could end in death. And they still make the gesture anyway because at that moment they are in such pain that they want to die, or at that moment, they are feeling impulsively self-destructive. They may be acting out homicidal anger toward another person by turning it inward unto themselves.

The fifth step is attempt. A patient like Courtney or Tiffany has survived a gesture and ended up in the ER. Now she has an idea of how much a fatal dosage might be. She drives alone up to a deserted mountain cabin and takes the presumed lethal dose.

The sixth step is suicide commission (death), an act of angry defiance, hopelessness, vengeful impulsivity, and self-loathing. There is often a sense of anger directed toward the survivors. This sixth degree can often be seen as an indictment of the people in the victim's life. It is by extension an indictment of that society in which they (we) all live. Most overdoses are not lethal, and of those, quite a few are not intended to be lethal by the overdoser. Gunshot to the head, however, is almost always lethal. People, who choose to overdose, might survive the first, second, and third overdose attempts. However, each time a person tries to overdose, she increases her risk of a fatal outcome. Males tend to use violent and lethal means such as hanging and guns. As a result, males are likelier to succeed in the first suicide attempt than women who have an apparent preference for intentional overdoses, and wrist cutting. This fact is reflected in the stories here: Jerrold, Derek, and Seth kill themselves on their first apparent attempt; Tiffany and Courtney survive; Matt intended to make only a gesture, but he made a serious judgment error that was fatal.

Suicide is a very bad decision for many reasons. At a basic level, a person may survive a suicide attempt but then be left in a vegetative state (in a nursing home) for the rest of his life. At a psychological level, suicide is a terminal form of displacing one's anger on to other persons or events, and is thus a toxic behavior. An unjust outcome might obtain under certain circumstances in which an innocent by-stander might be wrongly accused of murder in cases where he is somehow innocently associated with an intentional suicide. Even worse, an innocent bystander might be accidentally killed: this happened in LA in April 2010, for example, when a man intentionally crashed his car into a pole—he survived, but unfortunately, an unseen thirteen-year old girl was trapped between the car and pole; and, she did perish. And finally, most major religions are opposed to suicide for one or more reasons. Since we humans do not really know the actual spiritual repercussions of suicide, I believe that it should also be avoided on these grounds at all costs. Anecdotally, suicide might have additional legal repercussions in some societies. In Old England, for example, suicide was punished financially—all the properties and monies of a suicide went to the King as this represented all the future taxes owing the Crown, that the King could have collected, had the suicide lived out a normal lifespan.

Ultimately, Suicide is a case of Terminal Depression.

DEREK

Derek is an anesthesiologist (M.D.) who works in a Pain Clinic and runs a Methadone Clinic. He knew that addiction to certain narcotic drugs (Fentanyl and Sufentanyl) was the commonest psychological condition for his medical specialty and he had resisted that temptation at all costs. However, he began dating a young woman who was a "high-class" prescription-drug addict. He did not know that when he met her. He did not know that she had set him up as an easy target. She truly did like him as a person but loved pills, of which she required ever-increasing amounts. She had told Derek that she had well-controlled "minor depression" for which she was taking Effexor. She neglected to tell him about Ambien, Valium, Wellbutrin, Vicodin, and Dexedrine. This is not unusual. She kept her drug cravings under control so that he did not overtly suspect anything out of the ordinary. She was bright, spontaneous, funny, and sophisticated. She was the most fascinating woman he had ever known, and he became obsessed with her.

One evening after a gala event where they had both drunk too much, she introduced him to cocaine and its sex-enhancing effects. Against his better judgment, he used it—but only once. Three weeks later, she convinced him to try it again. Within a short time, he was using cocaine with her on a semi-regular basis. Then she introduced him to heroin. Not long after that, he began to crave heroin. And then she overdosed in his condo. He took her to the nearest ER where she was given medication treatment for narcotic overdose, but then she had seizures. She was sent up to the ICU where it was also determined that she had blood poising (septicemia) and bacterial heart disease (endocarditis) from multi-drug resistant *Staph. aureus* infection (MDRSA). She had heart and lung disease as well as uncontrolled seizure activity. Despite the best of efforts, she succumbed to all these medical problems (and died).

Derek had to answer many questions (from the police, medical board, and hospital) and had to deal with grief and his own incipient drug addiction. He felt very depressed and was grieving also. He was craving narcotics, so he started to snitch small amounts of methadone from his clinic. He needed more and more money to buy heroin and narcotics so he started to bill CMS (Medicare and Medicaid) with excessive (and fraudulent) claims for fictitious patients. CMS might eventually figure this out and punish him with multiple penalties. He was randomly called in for urine drug testing, and his urine was positive for narcotics. He lost his job at the Methadone Clinic and was placed under supervision at the Pain Clinic. Then he started sleeping with one of his patients who was taking a major narcotic, Dilaudid. She became angry when Derek's supervisor weaned her off Dilaudid, and Derek was unable to prescribe it for her (because his license had been restricted by the Medical Board). She started to blackmail him (for sleeping with her). His Depression really spiraled out of control when the investigators from the DOJ (Department of Justice) showed up one day. He bought a handgun and shot himself.

Discussion: Narcotics are very powerful drugs that can wreck a person's life. They cause a secondary Depression because they are "downers" for the nervous system. Toward the end of his life, Derek felt that everything he had worked for was in shambles. His medical license would be suspended, and his reputation, ruined. He also lost someone whom he loved—or thought that he loved. A visit by the DOJ would likely have led to hefty monetary fines and incarceration, not to mention that he would probably never again be able to see Medicare and Medicaid patients. He also knew that a number of anesthesiologists addicted to Fentanyl never achieve satisfactory recovery (overcoming Fentanyl is said to be much harder than beating alcoholism or Valium addiction). Physicians are better versed in the dangers of these drugs but this does not give them complete immunity from these sorts of problems. This is ultimately a case of Terminal Depression and Suicide of desperation.

Diagnosis: Reactive Depression, Grief, Secondary Depression due to Narcotics, and Suicide.

SETH

He is an outstanding student of science and math. Seth was very traditional in the sense that he still carried a briefcase to school and owned a slide rule which he knew how to operate. His friends and acquaintances were like-minded, although among them he really had no close friends, bosom buddies—partly because he always felt that he must compete with them and come out on top. He had met most of his high school friends in Astronomy club, Science club, and so on. He was always ahead of the rest of the class, and sometimes ahead of the teachers, too. This was a stable pattern throughout many years of school.

Despite his superb scholastic record, he seemed to be somewhat undecided about his future career goals, a trait perhaps typical of high schoolers, but less typical of high achievers. Maybe the best way to express this situation is that he appeared to have an "academic wanderlust." Or a certain emptiness. He also seemed to be seeking something that was apparently out of reach. Nobody was certain what this might be. Neither did he, apparently. Little was known about his home life or his siblings—or if he even had siblings. His friends were not invited to the house.

After graduating from high school, he went to Large State University where he did alright for a couple months but then he began to experience a great deal of unexpected emotional turmoil. He could not concentrate, his thoughts were racing, he felt even more socially disenfranchised than at any time in his life, which is to say, totally disenfranchised; and, for the first time in his life, he was feeling academically marginalized. He went to see his professors during their office hours, but the words coming out of his mouth seemed irrational and his thoughts seemed disconnected. This had never happened in high school where he was accustomed to being at or above the intellectual level of all the teachers.

He felt absolutely frantic day and night and could not sleep. He ended up taking himself to the Hospital ER on a very busy Saturday evening because of his intense inner agitation, but it was only an internal symptom. Outwardly, he looked relatively calm. The student doctors decided that he was neurotic and sent him home with several Valium pills. Seth took all the pills. He was calm for about twenty hours until the pills wore off, and then he tried to jump off the roof of his dorm but landed two stories below on the balcony of the Senior Resident Adviser who rounded up some freshmen and they forcibly carried Seth back— much to his utter humiliation—to the ER where the SRA insisted that Seth be admitted to the Psych Unit.

Somehow, Seth escaped the locked Psych Unit (possibly by defeating the electronic locking mechanism) and was trying to hang himself from a tree behind the hospital. But then a crowd of drunken students started jeering him on and he was so humiliated that he abandoned that attempt and went coursing back to his dorm room where he stood on his desktop and grabbed an opened can of ether that he had been keeping there for just such an occasion. The ether explosion killed Seth and rocked the dorm.

Discussion: These types of cases are puzzling, because the students are so gifted. One ominous possibility is that of a serious psychiatric illness which debuts in the late teens or early twenties. This could have been the beginning of Manic Depression or schizophrenia (as documented in the movie, *A Beautiful Mind*). Suicides occurring during the onset of Manic-Depression may be due to the Depression itself, or to Seth's realization that he is abnormal and feels that life is no longer of value. Remember, that these young men do not know that their Depression is just a phase of Manic-Depression that will eventually go away (for a while). Since they have never experienced this before, they may assume that this profound Depression is permanent—and they can not stand living in this new emotional state. The Depression itself might seem unbearable because it can present as a highly agitated Depression that is symptomatically very uncomfortable for the patient. There are other possibilities, including financial catastrophe at home or the burden of childhood emotional trauma. He may also have realized that he might not be the top science student in a huge university: the competition might have been intimidating—this can sometimes result in severe prolonged panic states; most people are not aware that untreated panic patients can have high suicide rates. Seth's suicide might have been related to any or all of these factors—or none.

Diagnosis: unknown ("Terminal Depression") suicide

Outcome: High school students should learn the basics of Depression in Health class so that they can help themselves and each other.

Matt: see Section on "Reactive Depression"
Jerrold: see his story under Depression associated with Child Abuse

PART THREE

TREATMENTS

People who see physicians (medical doctors) are called
"patients"

People who see all other mental health providers
(therapists, psychologists, counselors) are referred to as
"clients".

Introduction to All
Treatments

Terms in use in this book:

"depression" refers to the concept of sadness used in everyday speech

"depressed" means *"sad"*

"Depression" refers to the formal diagnosis of clinical Depression

"Depressed" means that the person has been diagnosed with clinical Depression

"Depressive" refers to the patient who has Depression

Many branches of Medicine are famous for having unusual treatments, and psychiatry is certainly no exception. Psychiatric treatments in general are all unusual and unique. The three well-known treatments are "talk therapy," powerful mood-stabilizing and mind-altering medications, and the notorious shock treatment (properly called ECT).

Of the three main treatments, the most unusual one is talk therapy which I am calling a social treatment, for the purposes of this book. This term highlights the fact that it is an intangible process based on personal interactions with another person, who is called the therapist or doctor. Few people realize this, but the therapist (or doctor) *is the treatment* and is the "delivery device" for this unique form of treatment. This interpersonal relationship may be one-on-one where the client spends nearly an hour with the therapist (or doctor). This is the "social" aspect of the treatment. Other variations of talk therapy may consist of two clients spending an hour with a therapist (marital therapy), or of a whole family spending time with a therapist (family therapy). Sometimes the social treatment may be that of a group of unrelated persons spending time with a therapist—or two therapists, if the group is large: this is group therapy.

Persons involved in a therapy group may have nothing in common and each person may be working on a number of different issues. This is general group therapy. In reality, even though most of these group members believe that they have different issues ("my boss", "my boyfriend", "my family") most of the participants are usually focusing on learning to interact more appropriately with other people—or learning how to be more mature and responsible ("my career goals"). There may be no one specific topic, other than learning how to relate better to others, in general.

However, many forms of group therapy nowadays focus on one specific issue. The group members identify themselves as having one narrowly focused problem and are all working on improving the way that they handle that one problem. Groups with such a specific problem (issue) may be men's groups, AA, anger management group, overweight/obesity, and so on. Some of these groups are formal and operate according to a time schedule, lasting only for a limited time span; and, a substantial fee may be charged for participation in these groups. These types of specific groups may follow other specific rules (these groups are often run by a hospital or are court-ordered). Other distinct kinds of specific groups are informal and lack both rules and leadership, and are nominally free of charge (AA and Alanon, for example). An intermediate type group may be run by large churches, which provide grief therapy, parents without partners, mixers for single church-members, and so on. Thus, talk therapy is social in the sense that it has an interpersonal aspect and does not involve manipulating the human body with chemicals (medications) or physical means (such as electricity, lights, magnetism, and so on).

The second unique psychiatric treatment is the use of medications that can cause major alterations in mood, thought, and behavior. Yes, it's true that your family doctor may prescribe you blood pressure pills that make you dizzy or kidney pills that cause increased urination, but psychiatric drugs are much more powerful in that they can change human behavior drastically, and the result of this can be drastic upheavals in governments and history. For example, Adolph Hitler was drugged up on massive amounts of amphetamines every day for years, drugs which can cause mania and psychosis. Not to mention many other historical leaders who were addicted to alcohol and opium. Not only are psychiatric medications very powerful drugs, but they can also be dangerous in the hands of non-psychiatrists. Many psychiatric drugs have "Black Box" warnings, which is a label assigned by the FDA (see Vocabulary) to drugs that can cause serious damage to the human body—or even death. Additionally, the DEA (see Vocabulary) also exerts strict controls over the distribution, prescribing, and dispensing of a number of psycho-active drugs. This is one reason that non-psychiatrists should not play around with these drugs, but, unfortunately, at least half of all psychiatric drugs are prescribed by non-psychiatrists. On the other hand, most of these medications prescribed to most people cause only subtle mood changes; but these subtle changes add up slowly over time, just like slowly accumulating any effect on a daily basis over the long-term.

The third unique treatment is ECT, vulgarly called "shock treatments." This is covered below in its own special section. ECT is actually very effective for very select patients. The shock can be delivered by electricity, insulin, or chemicals, but electricity is the only real delivery system in common use nowadays.

Other unique treatments in psychiatry include phototherapy (simulated sunlight), magnetic waves, and biofeedback.

Here is a list of these basic types of treatment:
I)-   Social: psychotherapy (talk therapy), counseling, group therapy, and residential placement (also called Milieu therapy)
II)-   Physical: exercise, biofeedback, electricity, light, and magnetism
III)-   Nutriceutics: Herbs, Hormones, Minerals, Vitamins, Food
IV)-   Pharmaceutics (Medications)
V)-   Therapeutics: the last topic in Part Three is *How to Find a Mental Health Provider*: I have mentioned this topic as a form of treatment because psychiatry is unique in that the provider is actually the Treatment, in the classical Freudian concept, at least.

I recommend starting with social treatments for mild cases. Medications can be added later, if necessary. For moderate cases, I recommend starting with at least two of the above three. Severe cases will definitely need medication from the outset and should include at least a few individual therapy sessions. Severe cases may also need Milieu treatment from the outset.

Ideal Treatment *Ideal treatment* is the treatment that results in significant improvement for the patient, which is an 85% improvement, by the standards of this book. Ideal treatment usually obtains when the treatment provided is the same treatment that would be provided by a random cross-section of a hundred psychiatrists, under the same circumstances. *Under-treatment* amounts to insufficient treatment to reach the 85% watermark. *Over-treatment* is prescribing excess treatment (too much medication, usually) that may approach 85%, but leaves the patient feeling overmedicated. *Improper treatment* is a treatment that lies outside the normal for both the majority of psychiatrists and for the "respected minority" of treating psychiatrists. (The "respected minority" may prescribe an old-fashioned or less popular treatment that nevertheless is acceptable treatment, just not the typical mainstream treatment— and, by definition, it also yields 85% improvement.) Improper treatment is typically delivered by family doctors and neurologists who often end up treating patients who absolutely refuse to see psychiatrists or who have no access to psychiatric care. *Self-treatment* occurs when the patient treats himself, and this can have very unpredictable outcomes. *Untreated*, of course, means that a Depression has been allowed to fester without any medical attention. In this case, the patient has refused to acknowledge the presence of a Depression; or, does acknowledge its presence, but refuses to see any doctor for treatment.

I)-Social Treatment

(Treatments without Chemicals)
Individual Psychotherapy, also simply called "Therapy"

These types of treatments involve an interpersonal activity, or connectivity, that acts indirectly on the mental and spiritual parts of the brain and not necessarily on the physical part of the brain as an organ of the body. However, intense sessions of therapy have been shown to have a temporary effect of increasing "feel-good" "brain hormones" for several hours thereafter. Social Treatments can be divided into individual therapy and counseling, as well as group therapy. Group therapy is available as formalized psychiatric groups or as informal self-help groups.

Social Treatment: Individual therapy
Overview
Individual therapy is also called talk therapy or psychotherapy. Professionals who deliver individual therapy may have either a master's degree or a doctorate. Individual therapy is oftenest undertaken with a therapist who typically has a master's degree. There are several designations at this level, such as Master's degrees in Marriage and Family Therapy, Licensed Clinical Social Worker, and so on (depending upon the State of licensure). Most psychotherapists have their own favored way of doing therapy, so Meg will need to ask about the particular bent of her new therapist on the first visit. Some therapists specialize on certain problem areas, such as marital therapy, long-term treatment of borderline syndrome, gay and lesbian issues, sex therapy, and so on. The training of therapists consists of a few years of general education followed by specialized education. The final phase of training consists

of working under the supervision of an experienced therapist—this is like an internship.

Psychotherapy may also be provided by various types of professionals holding doctorate degrees: psychologists (Ph.D.), clinical psychologists (Psy.D.), and others. Psychologists are doctors of psychology (Ph.D.) who have training in academics, research, and psychological testing; and, they are also providers of individual psychotherapy. Clinical psychologists hold a doctorate, Psy.D. Their training has focused mainly on doing psychotherapy with clients. Earning these types of doctorates takes longer than earning a master's degree, so therapy with these doctorate level professionals can be expected to cost more. (These types of doctors are not medical doctors.) There are also a few other doctorate degrees which permit practicing individual therapy on a limited basis.

Additionally, there are medical doctors, M.D. and D.O. These doctors are referred to as psychiatrists—not psychologists. Psychiatrists may provide psychotherapy, but that is not very common nowadays. If they do so, it is usually an abbreviated form of therapy that may conclude with the writing or changing of prescriptions, based on the information gleaned during the therapy session. The main roles of most modern psychiatrists are to prescribe treatment (usually in the form of medications), order pertinent lab tests, and to interface with family doctors, neurologists, and other medical doctors who might be involved directly in the care of the patient. Other types of psychiatric prescriptions may include physical treatments (that act directly on the body) such as electrical waves (ECT), magnetic waves (tCMR), light waves (photo-therapy), and so on.

Finally, psycho-analysts are psychiatrists (medical doctors) who have undergone a very lengthy training period in order provide psycho-analysis (like Sigmund Freud). There are very few of these doctors, and their services can be very costly.

Talk Therapy

"Talk Therapy" (individual psychotherapy) is an important part of the treatment process. Numerous studies have documented that some patients experience 50% relief from psychotherapy alone, and that some patients derive 50% benefit from medications alone. The possibility of feeling really good is often achievable by combining an appropriate amount of psychotherapy sessions along with the judicious use of psychiatric medicines. This combination has been estimated to yield 75-85% improvement, based on similar studies. This is the basis upon which I state my sincere belief that 85% of patients can feel 85% better if they follow the complete treatment plan that I prescribe. Individual psychotherapy (talk therapy) with a therapist or psychologist will serve a twofold purpose of being confessional and stress-lowering, which has been demonstrated by changes in levels of biochemical markers in the body. The whole treatment process can be somewhat complicated but only for a minority of people. Most people will have a very unremarkable experience. Anything that seems remarkable at first will have been—in hindsight—probably due to the initial anxiety of the client/patient.

Therapeutic Alliance
This will hopefully materialize in the first few sessions of therapy (typically with a therapist or psychologist). This is a condition in which both the therapist and the client feel that the relationship is workable and can be therapeutic. This relationship will hopefully continue until the client feels better.

Ongoing Therapy
This is the period of time (weeks, months, years) during which therapy continues on a regular basis. The length of time in treatment will depend upon several factors. If a person has a persistent and serious problem (incest and sexual abuse), then the length of treatment may be very long. Patients with less serious problems may require shorter treatment times, such as one or two years. Some people may stay until they feel better, and then quit therapy to see if they can continue to feel good without it. They may return to therapy in the future if they feel the need for more. Duration of treatment can be discussed during the phase of ongoing therapy.

Termination of Therapy
This refers to that time when the client, Meg, would like to stop having regular appointments with the doctor or therapist. Meg will eventually arrive at a point where the therapy is not anticipated to provide much more immediate benefit. This can be mutually discussed with the

therapist and a course of action can be decided. Usually the therapy will not be terminated abruptly, but will slowly be phased out and then there will come the last session. At this point, Meg will start to rely upon herself, being armed with what she has learned about herself in therapy. She will learn to use community resources and other available sources. Of course, she is free to leave the therapy relationship whenever she chooses, but it should be announced in advance in case the therapist or doctor wish to give cautionary feedback.

And when this whole talk therapy process is finished and she is able to have a mutual termination, then she is ready to make a "flight into health" to see how well she can "fly" on her own. If not doing so well, then she can always come back for more therapy.

If Meg has chosen treatment that includes both talk therapy and medication, then the psychiatrist will prescribe and monitor any needed medications while talk therapy progresses. If the medications are helpful, she may choose to continue the medications even after the therapy sessions have come to an end; this plan should be discussed with the doctor.

Social Treatment: Counseling

Another form of individual attention is for a client to have regular sessions with a counselor. For example, alcohol counselors have typically gone through a similar—but shorter—training period than that of therapists; apart from fulfilling their general education requirements, they may have additional year(s) of specialized education and one year (2,000 hours in California) of supervised "internship." Counselors usually have a narrow focus of interest, such as alcohol counseling.

Social Treatment: Group Therapy

Group Therapy refers to any therapy done by two or more clients/ participants. Group therapy can be subdivided into formalized therapy groups and informal groups. The formalized groups are psychologically focused and are run by a mental health professional who will charge each member per session (perhaps $25-40). Informal groups, such as Twelve Steps programs, have no oversight from mental health professionals, have no real leadership, and are basically free of cost. Regardless of type or focus of the group, all groups are intended to provide support for people in difficult situations. Groups can also offer a sense of hope by providing exposure to other people who are on the same path, so that apparent pain can be shared and not borne alone.

Formalized group therapy is run by mental health professionals, who are sometimes referred to as facilitators; these groups may have one specific focus or may have a general focus. Examples of groups with a specific focus are men's groups, anger management groups, incest survivors groups, DUI diversion programs, and so on. Formalized therapy groups with a general focus usually revolve around the group members' concerns about their personal psychological issues. These groups also help members face the problems they experience in interacting with other people in general. In this sense, the general-focus group can give valuable insight and feedback to group members who are trying to understand how their personality styles undermine their relationships with other people. Thus, the group operates as a "mini-community" in which the participants can learn from their peers how other people perceive them. These groups are run by a mental health professional who tries to help the group focus on one issue, one member's issues, or one topic at a time. The mental health professional intervenes when feedback or criticism from other group-members becomes harsh or when the group strays off-track. This type of therapy is especially helpful for people who have trouble seeing themselves as they really are—that includes a lot of us! These groups will cost some money, which pays the mental health facilitator ("referee"). After these specific groups have finished, participants may be encouraged to continue recovery by joining informal problem-specific groups such as A.A., A.C.A (Adult Children of Alcoholics), E.A. (Emotionals Anonymous), D.A. (Debtors Anonymous), and so on.

At a more informal level are the problem-specific groups such as Twelve Steps programs which offer members a specific type of therapy with a narrow focus of interest. These groups have no formalized leadership and are established to help people suffering from severe compulsive behaviors. The people who establish these groups also suffer from the same specific problems that the groups are designed to address. There is a tradition of changing "leadership," although there is no real leadership—merely "suggestions." The mutual support in these groups is usually more extensive than in formal groups: the advantage of this is that more support is reliably available between meetings, but the disadvantage is that groups members can become embroiled in each other's personal issues. On the bright side, Twelve Steps programs cost almost nothing—a nominal one-dollar donation at each meeting. It is generally recognized that attendance at these meetings has no time limit and may continue for years and decades, perhaps indefinitely, which serves to reinforce the community spirit of continuity. The original Twelve Step program was Alcoholics Anonymous (A.A.). This was followed by Alanon which is for the family members of alcoholics. After that came Narcotics Anonymous (N.A.), and other programs such as O.A. (Overeaters Anonymous), E.A, (Emotionals Anonymous for psychological problems), D.A. (Debtors Anonymous), S.L.A.A. (Sex and Love Addicts Anonymous), G.A. (Gamblers Anonymous), and others (focusing on Crystal Meth, Cocaine, Marijuana, and so on).

Other types of group therapy include marital therapy, couples therapy, family therapy, sex therapy, and so on.

If you are just embarking on a course of treatment and have a lot of doubts, remember that if you drop out, then your misery might come back again. You may take one step forward and half a step backward and may feel very frustrated and unhappy. You are in this for the full treatment, and you should not quit mid-way. Remember the old saying "quitters never win, and winners never quit." And most importantly, as you go along, try to remember that

"Pain may be necessary, but suffering is optional."

Everybody wants to get better and feel better, but some group patients may appear so disorganized that they cannot focus on treatment and may appear to sabotage their own treatment by not following through with treatment goals. If they can stay in treatment until the fog lifts, then they too can get on track and "make a flight into health."

Social Treatment: Residential Placement, Milieu Therapy
("Milieu" is French for "[treatment] center")
This type of treatment refers to a closed environment or a social setting. The closed—or enclosed—environment is typically separated from the outside world by well-defined boundaries. The boundaries may be invisible, loosely enforced, or very concrete. The loosest boundaries

would be those of designating the last six rooms on a hospital ward for a certain condition, such as for patients requiring a medical "detox" (detoxification from alcohol and drugs). In another case, one whole ward of a hospital might be separated by an unlocked door from other wards on the same floor—this might be set aside for a 28-day drug and alcohol program. A more isolated version may be that of a freestanding residence that houses half a dozen very disabled patients with Bipolar Depression. Patients who have a Severe Depression may need to be placed involuntarily into a locked psychiatric ward. Psychotic Depression may require hospitalization in order to begin a course of shock treatments, which will require a few weeks to complete. Anyone who is suicidal also needs to be in a psychiatric hospital for a minimum of seventy-two hours of observation. Patients with difficult-to-treat (treatment-refractory) Manic Depression may need to be sent to a long-term State mental hospital.

Depressed Dementia patients may also be hospitalized for a short period of time—perhaps in a locked geriatric ward of the hospital. If these elderly patients with dementia also have a psychotic Depression, then they will be stabilized on a geriatric ward and then transferred for long-term confinement in a locked nursing home—or a nursing home that has one locked unit for such patients.

Recovery homes are another example of Milieu setting. These sites have been established to help recovering alcoholics and addicts like Rhonda. The length of stay could be as short as a month or as long as a year or more. Depressed alcoholics and addicts often require more recovery time than recovering alcoholics and addicts without Depression (or other major psychiatric diagnoses). Rhonda needs milieu placement because she has two major disorders: Addiction and Secondary Depression. And, the worse the Depression, the more time is required to recover. (Mild depression will have a shorter recovery time than a severe Depression.) Rhonda has the frustrated feeling of trying to control two diseases simultaneously: Depression and Addiction. She can spend many months or years trying to get them both under control, but at least in her case, only a year was required (because she had only a mild Secondary Depression).

It is extremely rare nowadays for people to be sent to a long-term psychiatric hospital. This setting is hugely costly and is available only to the very wealthy or to severely ill patients who are already in the county or state systems.

Other residential placement could involve transfer to an unlocked nursing home-type environment for short-term care or long-term care or to a Board-and-Care setting.

II)-Physical Treatment

Physical Treatment involves some physical activity that acts directly on the brain as a physical organ of the body. These beneficial physical activities may be exercise and biofeedback. A subset of physical treatment includes so-called biophysical treatments involving the use of mechanically induced physical forces (electricity, light, and magnetism) to cause beneficial reactions in the brain. Since these latter treatments act on the body and are "invasive," technically speaking, they must be prescribed by a medical doctor. (The licenses of MD/DO psychiatrists are legally described as "license to practice Medicine and Surgery in the State of _____.")

Exercise: These treatment techniques are usually in the form of daily aerobics, meditation, yoga, and such. These kinds of activities can release our natural internal "narcotics" and other feel-good "brain hormones." And no, these natural "brain narcotics" will not cause relapse in Rhonda who is a recovering narcotics addict. These chemicals are already in our brains. Although they might provide pleasurable feelings after aerobics, they are not addicting in the same sense as are narcotic drugs, such as heroin.

Biofeedback (BFB): This is a technique of self-control which can be quickly learned by using a BFB machine. This machine "teaches" the patient how to control his pulse and blood pressure, thereby allowing him to remain serene in the presence of great stress or anxiety. If a patient has no access to a BFB machine, then this technique can gradually be acquired by prolonged use of guided insight-meditation.

Sunlight

Another kind of Physical Treatment is phototherapy for Winter Depression. This is a special light-box with full spectrum light bulbs that are like natural sunlight. Not surprisingly, sunlight has been shown to have a mild antidepressant effect. Phototherapy is quite effective for Winter Depression, but can be used for any mild Depression, too. Darkness (nighttime) stimulates the pineal gland to secrete melatonin, another natural "brain hormone." Melatonin naturalizes and regularizes our twenty-four hour cycle. Likewise, extra sunlight is thought to have positive benefits on our twenty-four hour cycle which is related to sleep cycles: sleep better, feel better.

Magnetism

The treatment is properly called Trans-Cranial Magnetic Resonance Therapy, a new technology that allows psychiatrists to send focused magnetic waves to the front of the brain for half an hour. This is a new treatment for moderate Depression. It is often effective. The patient may have a temporary headache after the treatment.

Electricity

And of course, the most famous—and infamous—psychiatric treatment is the so-called "shock treatment." Our name for shock treatment is ECT (Electro-Convulsive Therapy).

An epileptic seizure (in the brain) can counteract the symptoms of severe Depression. The reason for this beneficial result is unknown, but ECT is known to cause a surge-release of dopamine and probably of other "feel-good" "anti-depressant brain hormones," too. Doctors have learned to deliver this kind of seizure artificially to Depressed patients (who do not suffer from epilepsy). People have vulgarly called this "shock treatment," based on the assumption that it is a shock [to the nervous system]. The technology for delivering ECT has greatly advanced over the last seventy years. ECT is now a safe therapy (except in certain brain diseases and after heart attacks).

The patient preparation involves placing one electrode on the right side of the head and another on the left-central side of the forehead The technique involves sending a brief pulse of electrical current between the two electrodes positioned on the front of the head, such that the pulse will travel through the brain. With modern technology, the seizure is isolated to the brain and does not spread to the rest of the body (such as heart and uterus), thus it is a safe treatment during pregnancy and in most heart patients. It is helpful in most Severe Depressions; however, because of the possibility of mild memory loss, its use nowadays is reserved for very select cases of Severe Depression that have not responded to all the usual medications, representing perhaps fewer than 0.01% of the entire Depressed population. ECT can also be used on an emergency basis so that patients will improve very quickly—in some cases, a faster recovery than with all the other treatments listed here in Part Three.

When ECT was first done in the middle of the last century, it earned a well-deserved bad reputation for being a horrible ordeal. It caused broken bones, memory loss, and loosened teeth. This is no longer a problem with modern technology. Nonetheless, there was great public outcry, and County and State governments removed it from their list of preferred treatments. ECT tends to be more expensive than most medications and is an excellent treatment for select cases. The real irony nowadays is that ECT is accessible only to those with exceptionally good health insurance. Some patients respond dramatically to ECT. In fact, some of these patients come in once a month for a "booster" dose of ECT.

Interesting factoids: (1) since ECT releases a surge of dopamine, patients with slowed motion from Parkinson's disease will also improve after ECT—but only for a while. (2) ECT is technically classified as surgery because it is invasive.

III)-"Nutriceutics"

Treatments with Herbs,
Hormones, Minerals, and Vitamins

Nutriceutics: Using nutritional and nature-sourced found substances as pharmaceuticals

Herbs in General

In America, **herbs** are defined as any therapeutic chemicals found in plants. Many people jump to the conclusion that herbs are better than man-made (synthetic) medications because they occur in nature. This is not true for many reasons. Firstly, the herbal product is usually a dried plant or a dried plant part. In other words, the whole leaf (or whole root or entire flowers) may be dried and powdered and then presented as an herbal treatment. A whole plant part such as a leaf contains hundreds of different chemicals, in the same sense that a human finger contains thousands of chemicals. The leaf is not one purified chemical. A person who eats the whole leaf may absorb the antidepressant chemical in the leaf, but he is also eating hundreds of other plant chemicals that might cause side effects. Secondly, we need to consider the growing conditions of the plant-herb: it might have grown in poor soil or rich soil; it might have had too much rain or not enough, too much sun and heat, or not enough, and so on. All of these changes in growing conditions alter the percentages of herbal-chemicals in the plant. Stunted plants might contain the same dose of antidepressant chemical regardless of the weight of the plant, but if the plant were badly stunted and grew to only half size, then this could represent a double concentration in a severely stunted plant; thus, the herbal product has a double dose of antidepressant per tablet. Sometimes the plant might have been grown in artificial chemical fertilizer or in soils heavy with metals or fields that receive runoff from animal grazing—the animals might be given daily doses of steroids, antibiotics, and other chemicals, all of which can trickle down into the herb plot. Thirdly, when the herb was harvested, maybe some undesirable weeds were collected along with the herbal plant and were admixed; perhaps the herb-harvest included some plants that had grown from seeds of GMO-plants (Genetically Modified Organisms) that had accidentally blown over from a nearby field. Maybe unscrupulous sellers of cheap herbal products deliberately (and illegally) mixed in other plant substances (like caffeine or ephedrine) to make the antidepressant effect seem stronger. When the FDA or designated agencies have spot-checked the quality of certain herbs, there have been significant variations in the amount of desirable chemicals in different lots of herb from different herbal companies—far greater variations than in synthetic medications.

Furthermore, a number of our man-made (synthetic) pharmaceuticals have been based on naturally occurring herbal products. So these synthetic medications are essentially natural: Nature-inspired but Factory-sourced. We make them in a factory because it is cheaper; and in this way, we can guarantee the purity of the chemical in the medication and the exact amount of medication in each pill. As the reader can discern, "natural" is not necessarily better after all.

HERB: ST. JOHN'S WORT (SJW)

The one commonly used antidepressant herb is **St John's Wort** (SJW) which can sometimes produce success in the treatment of Depression where several synthetic drugs have failed. It can also interact with synthetic medications, especially synthetic antidepressants. SJW can also cause birth defects if taken during pregnancy. St John's Wort contains more than one chemical with antidepressant properties, and these can all vary in percentages in relation to each other, also. For example, hypericin is considered to be the active ingredient in SJW, and it can vary from 0.3%-0.4%; hyperforin also adds some antidepressant properties to SJW and it can vary 2-4% (data from A. José Lança MD PhD). If we look at the quality-control parameters for Prozac manufacture, the amount of fluoxetine in every Prozac capsule is identical in dosage and purity and does not vary because of weather, nearby cow-grazing, and so on.

A few other herbs are used in psychiatry such as valerian and kava, both of which may help anxiety.

Hormones: None of these hormones are intended for long-term use in Depression. None of them are used as primary treatment of Depression or are even FDA-approved for Depression. Their only use is as an add-on to the usual antidepressants and mood-stabilizing medications, and to be used only for a couple months to energize a sluggish Depression. Although the hormones are not FDA-approved, some of them may be used in response to low blood levels of these hormones, a sometimes-frequent finding in Depression. Cytomel has been used routinely by Depression experts, and a fair amount of information exists about this use, most of it inconclusive.

Thyroid hormone: (Cytomel) is sometimes used as an add-on treatment in treating Chronic Depression, Recurrent Unipolar Depression, or Depressed patients who are taking Lithium. Cytomel can help a person to feel somewhat more animated and activated. Low thyroid blood levels may often be caused by the Depression itself, and when the Depression is well-treated, the thyroid levels may renormalize, thus eliminating any justification for using Cytomel. Since Lithium can alter thyroid hormone levels, there may or may not be any justification for using Cytomel in these patients—and certainly not for long-term use. If thyroid hormone blood levels remain too low for too long, then the Lithium-treated patient should be sent to an endocrinologist. Orally available thyroid hormones include T4 (thyroxine) and T3 (Cytomel), as well as Thyrolar™ (of natural bovine source).

"Male Hormones": can sometimes make elderly men feel more animated, but this effect is variable. Most of my patients who have tried this as an add-on treatment do not find it helpful in the long-term and stop it after a month or two. Besides, these hormones are not suitable for long-term use as they can cause many biological problems. Some men with chronic diseases (such as HIV/AIDS) may benefit from this treatment. This treatment may take the form of "male hormones" (testosterone) or anabolic hormones (derivatives of "male hormones"), such as oxandrolone and others.

Growth Hormone (GH): has been used for performance-enhancement and may produce a sense of well-being. Currently, GH has no recognized treatment benefits for Depression.

Hormone: Melatonin: see above under Physical Treatment, Sunlight.

MINERAL: LITHIUM

There is one mineral that is used as a mood stabilizer, although it is not a true antidepressant. This is lithium, which is a "natural" treatment because it is a mineral (an alkali earth salt, to be exact). Lithium is mined in open salt pits (in North Carolina and Bolivia, for example). Lithium salts are hauled to a laboratory where the lithium is "purified" [extracted] and combined with carbonic acid or citric acid (both are "natural" organic acids that exist abundantly in nature and in our bodies). People may take lithium carbonate or lithium citrate: the carbonate is a powder suitable for tablets and capsules, whereas the citrate provides a liquid form of lithium that can be drunk. Carbonate is the chemical in baking powder and baking soda; citrate (and citric acid) come from citrus fruits. Lithium is in the same chemical family as sodium and potassium, which are common minerals. Sodium and potassium are very abundant in every cell in our bodies and are essential for life as we know it. Lithium does not normally occur in our body or at least, not in any measurable amount; therefore, the normal blood level of lithium is zero. This "natural" treatment can cause very serious side effects if its blood levels double. In other words, if a patient's lithium blood level increases from 1.2 to 2.4, he can have very, very serious medical problems. Lithium may be "natural" but it is also naturally poisonous at double dose. Anyone taking Lithium needs close medical supervision.

Vitamin-D is increasingly being shown to be important in numerous medical conditions; this is not surprising, since it is dependent on natural sunlight, which is believed to have mild antidepressant effects.

"VITAMINS" (THESE ARE BOTH REALLY AMINO ACIDS)

SAM-e (S-Adenosyl Methionine) is a derivative of the amino acid methionine which occurs naturally as one of the building blocks of proteins; methionine occurs throughout the human body. SAM-e seems to have some antidepressant properties; however, there are few data on the safety of using SAM-e medicinally on a long-term basis.

L-Tryptophan is an amino acid used by our bodies to produce serotonin, the antidepressant "brain hormone," which is a normal part of our brain biochemistry. L-Tryptophan at bedtime helps promote sleep (in dosages of three to five grams); when combined with certain antidepressants (Trazodone), L-Tryptophan can boost the antidepressant effect. And no, unfortunately, a diet rich in L-Tryptophan does not of itself prevent or cure Depression.

Diet: Food is one of our main contacts with the physical world. Food is fuel and nutrient, building blocks of health, and in a sense it is also medication. Foods certainly are the mortar and bricks that are used to patch up our time-weary bodies. Vegetables rich in vitamins and minerals are a kind of herbal treatment. Fruits may be included, too. Dairy products are a protein source. Chinese peapods contain dopamine. Many proteins contain the amino acid, Tryptophan, a precursor of serotonin. Dopamine and serotonin are the anti-depressant "brain hormones" necessary for making us feel good. Other foods are sources of other vitamins, minerals, trace elements, and the so-called "essential amino acids," which are amino acids that cannot be made inside our bodies and must be acquired from external sources. The right kinds of food are important, but it is also important to remember to control our physical contact with them in order to avoid becoming overweight.

Many people eat large amounts of junk food and fast food which have non-nutritious chemicals such as table salt, common sugar, fats, and chemicals of all sorts. We all know that table salt raises blood pressure which can then cause high blood pressure and kidney stress; sugar causes diabetes and obesity; and, fats cause obesity. Even worse are all the chemicals, such as BHT, EDTA, pyrogallate, and all the food-dyes with such unappetizing names as FD&C·#5. We used EDTA in our college chemistry labs and it never once crossed my mind to swill some down before adding it to acetone. A lot of the food-dyes are related to very toxic substances. I do not understand why people insist on consuming these harmful chemicals. One of the greatest public health measures occurred in our country when the government required all prepared and processed foods to list ingredients and calories in the boxed "Nutrition Facts" printed on all these foodstuffs. This information seemingly goes unheeded by most people—to their detriment.

IV)-Pharmaceutical Treatment

Prescription Medications
(Drugs of Pharmaceutical Quality)

There are many kinds of prescription medications used in treatment of Depression. Four different types of medications may be employed: primary antidepressants, secondary medications, mood stabilizers, and side effect pills. The primary antidepressants are the main treatment for Depression. There are also some secondary medications that possess mild antidepressant properties or that help the antidepressants work more smoothly. The third level of treatment is that of mood stabilizers which are often useful for Cycling Depressions (those that are characterized by up and down moods). There is also a small group of side-effect medications which are prescribed to treat any unpleasant side effects related to the use of the other three types of medications. The secondary medications and side effect pills can be deployed in cases where Marc or Meg feel very well with their primary antidepressant treatment—except for one little nagging side effect. (this book covers only the primary antidepressants—the other three classes are discussed in *Defeating Depression*). As you may guess, the formalized treatment of a serious Major Depression might indeed require a primary antidepressant, a secondary medication, plus a side-effect pill. Many people like Altagràcia or Carrie-Beth might balk at so many medicines, but that is simply where our technology has taken us up to this point. If she does not wish to take any prescription medications, then doctors cannot legally force her to do so, unless her life is in immediate jeopardy.

A different situation may occur with some patients like Louise who may try several antidepressants, not one of which provides optimal relief. These are the possible explanations:

- Louise did not take the individual pills for long enough or at high/low enough doses;
- she does not have a biochemical Depression;
- she has a biochemical Depression, but there is no medication available that will give her relief—in other words, the antidepressant that she needs may not yet exist;
- maybe her diagnosis should be reviewed;
- she should look into a non-pharmacological treatment such as talk therapy, light therapy, magnetism, or herbs; or,
- she needs a longer time to respond to any antidepressant—for reasons as yet unknown, but this can happen.

I have had Depressed patients who have tried a few medications sequentially (each one for about six weeks), and then finally after some months, have rather suddenly started to have a robust response to the next antidepressant that they try. Either this is a really good medication, or the many medications already taken, "primed the pump" for the next antidepressant, regardless of which antidepressant it is. This is an example of the observation that some people need to be treated for lengthy periods before they have a really great response. Perhaps, if they had stayed on the first antidepressant for six months continuously, then they might have finally had a great response—but we have no instruments or lab tests to predict this outcome. In the real world, it is difficult to get patients to take the same apparently "useless" medication for six months while having no response, but while awaiting a response. Patients know that there are many choices of antidepressants available, and they want to jump to the next one. Moreover, this is not how modern psychiatrists practice: we do not favor keeping a person on an apparently useless drug for six months, because we also know that there are many untried choices. Furthermore, keeping a patient on this same medicine for six months while awaiting a possible response would be out of line with the "usual and customary" practice of modern psychiatry. By extension, it could even be viewed as unethical.

A trial of six weeks is often considered an adequate trial of a [non-helpful] medication. Often the medication will or will not exert its effect between weeks two and four—this is a fairly routine happenstance.

After week four, if there is no response, a change of medications or the use of an add-on drug ("weak" antidepressant) may be contemplated. If there is no response by week six, then a change in medication tactics is definitely in order. The worse dilemma is what to do if Louise starts to have a response at three weeks as predicted, but she only feels about 40% better. There are a number of tactics for dealing with this situation. Another thorny problem occurs when she has responded well to the antidepressant around the third week and is feeling great until week eight or nine at which time the effect seems to be fading. These are complicated cases, and these are the ones who are referred from primary care doctors to psychiatrists. Sometimes in these cases, minor interventions may be helpful, and sometimes, an extensive treatment overhaul is indicated. Once again, I repeat that Louise should go see a psychiatrist. I do not say this to make business good, but because I see too many people who have waited too long, resisted help, and come to the office in a significantly deteriorated state that could have been completely avoided by a timely intervention: better sooner than later. Louise suffers more, and it makes my job more difficult: same situation in which you decide not to change the oil in your car for thirty thousand miles because you do not want to spend the money. Better to have too much treatment than not enough.

There are a few medications which are known to have a lag time to onset. Nardil is exactly such a drug. It almost always takes effect between weeks five and six. When Nardil was popular, I would usually schedule return visits of Nardil patients at two, four and six weeks. Weeks two and four were for the "pep talk" to encourage a patient to keep taking it despite lack of any apparent response. On week six, my Nardil patients showed up feeling good and optimistic and sometimes a bit flushed. There is no reason not to assume that other medications might have similar effects in some patients. Tincture of Time and Potion of Patience.

Our ability to tolerate antidepressant medications is rooted in our genetics. You may be unable to tolerate certain antidepressants: this is not your imagination. In other cases, you may be able to tolerate antidepressants, but you end up needing very high doses or only very low doses of the antidepressants. This also is your genetics at work behind the scenes (in your liver and brain). This is a real effect due to genetics and is explained in great detail in my book, *Everyone's Everyday Guide to Practical Psychiatry* (Section II-4).

TREATMENT STRATEGY

The theoretical considerations involved in choosing an antidepressant rely on an attempt to try to balance the patient's needs in regards to his presenting symptoms, while taking into account how he might like to feel. Psychiatrists balance many factors while trying to make the best medication choice for each patient (this is explained in detail in my book, *Defeating Depression*). This following list of medications represents facts that are only approximations of what to expect in real clinical practice—every person has unique chemistry and unique responses to the medications.

LISTS OF MEDICATIONS
AND
RELEVANT TERMS

The following list includes most antidepressants in current use in the USA. Some of the medications on the list are rarely used today, but are included for the sake of completeness. This list *does not* include the secondary medications, mood stabilizers, or the side effect pills (see my first two books). Certain terms relevant to medication usage are also included. The complete list of terms, abbreviations, and definitions appears at the very end of the book.

ANTIDEPRESSANT MEDICATIONS

Amoxapine—see Asendin

Amitriptyline—this is generic Elavil; when this generic form first became available, some patients complained that it did not seem the same as brand-name Elavil; this has not been reported as a problem in later years; see Elavil

Amphetamines—see Stimulants

Anafranil—is a potent tricyclic antidepressant with anti-obsessive properties. Apart from that, its side effects can be read in the Tricyclic section below; generic name: clomipramine

Antidepressants in general can cause dry mouth, nervousness, insomnia. Some antidepressants are used to treat ADHD as well as Depression: for example, Effexor, Imipramine, Strattera, Wellbutrin, and the stimulant antidepressants such as Ritalin and various amphetamine salts; there is more on this topic following this list.

Asendin—is a tricyclic (generic Amoxapine), but is also closely related to an antipsychotic medication, Loxitane. Asendin has milder side effects than the [other] tricyclics. However, it can cause Parkinsonism which is often permanent. Its use should be restricted to psychiatrists only.

Atomoxetine (SNRI antidepressant used for ADHD)—see Strattera

"BRAIN HORMONE"—refers to the various bio-chemicals in the brain that regulate behavior and mood, the three most important of which are dopamine, serotonin, and norepinephrine; see Vocabulary at end of book

BRAND-NAME / BRANDED MEDICATIONS, PATENT MEDICINES, TRADE-NAME MEDICATIONS: these four terms all refer to the original medications which were first marketed by the parent drug company before the seventeen year patent expired, after which generic versions of the branded drug could be sold; see this topic in Vocabulary at end of book

Bupropion—see Wellbutrin

Celexa—this is an SSRI antidepressant. For its side effects, see SSRI's. Celexa may be less likely to cause serious "discontinuation syndrome." Some people require higher doses of Celexa, and the HMO insurance plans are very reluctant to authorize this (extra expense). Fortunately, Celexa is now available in a less expensive generic form. Celexa is available in an alcohol-free liquid form and also in a "purified" version called Lexapro. See Lexapro.

Citalopram—see Celexa

Clomipramine—see Anafranil

Cylert—currently off the market in USA; this is a stimulant antidepressant that is less addicting than Ritalin and the amphetamines. It has a very small role in treatment of childhood ADHD and can be used in certain forms of Depression. It may stress the liver. It has caused liver failure in very isolated cases.

Cymbalta—is an SSNRI which means that it acts on serotonin and norepinephrine, both of which are presumed to have natural antidepressant activity inside our brain. Cymbalta is also approved for use in diabetic nerve pain (and may be a helpful non-addictive treatment for other chronic pains). (compare to Effexor)

Desipramine—see Norpramin

Desvenlafaxine—see Pristiq/Effexor

Desyrel—is a multi-purpose antidepressant related to Serzone (and Buspar) that is so frequently used, that it is usually called by its generic name, Trazodone. Its original function was as a calmative antidepressant to be given twice or more per day. It has found its "market niche," however, as a sleeping pill for patients who are mildly Depressed and who have trouble sleeping; even more commonly it is used as a secondary medication with the SSRI and SSNRI antidepressants either as a secondary antidepressant or as a sleeping aid; it is very popular with psychiatrists. Most patients who take it, report good success; a few people stop taking Desyrel because it makes them dizzy or nauseous; it is best absorbed with a very small carbohydrate snack, but if a person is on a strict diet, then she can take a slightly higher dose. It should not be used in men who are still sexually potent since it can cause priapism which becomes a medical emergency that—in extremely rare cases—can result in permanent impotence: I discuss this with male patients, and no one wants to take it except for those men who are permanently impotent from diabetes, prostate surgery, or who have had a penis removed for penile cancer. I had one female patient who reported clitoral discomfort—I have prescribed it to thousands of women without any other such reports; Desyrel *must not* be prescribed in cases of severe heart problems called ventricular arrhythmias; Trazodone blood levels are available, but are rarely necessary; Trazodone does not cause cataracts as once thought (the early research had been done with beagles who are well known to develop cataracts naturally);

Dexedrine—was one of the first antidepressants ever invented; in recent decades, this antidepressant has become popular as a treatment for ADHD; it is available in several sizes as well as timed release preparations— see Stimulants

Dextro-amphetamine—see Dexedrine and Stimulant antidepressants

DISCONTINUATION SYNDROME—see SSRI

Doxepin—see Sinequan

DRUG—refers to "street drug," addicting medication, or illegal drug (in this book)

Duloxetine—see Cymbalta

ECT—Electro-Convulsive Treatment, treatment for severe Depression typically using electricity ("shock treatment")—in the past, certain chemicals and insulin were also used to induce a "shock" (a brain seizure)

Effexor—is an SSNRI medication which is active on serotonin at lower doses and active on both serotonin and norepinephrine at higher doses; this range of biochemical activity improves Depression; this range of effects also makes Effexor effective for decreasing nerve pain and chronic pain; Effexor is an excellent treatment for adult ADHD, and in all ADHD cases where addicting psycho-stimulants should not be used; it has a few side effects such as headaches and dizziness, but these usually disappear after the first or second week of treatment; Effexor can also cause constipation;

Effexor can aggravate high blood pressure or even cause high blood pressure which is sometimes difficult to control even with blood pressure pills; Effexor can also cause discontinuation syndrome; Effexor is available in rapid-release tablets and delayed-release capsules; another common side effect (mainly with the tablets) is stomach irritation which can be treated with "Histamine/H$_2$ blockers" (Pepcid, Axid); Effexor is now available in a "purified" version, Pristiq;

Elavil—is one of the tricyclics; it has been used for many psychiatric, neurological, and medical purposes, including but not limited to: Depression, anxiety, insomnia, migraines, and chronic pain; It has all the usual tricyclic antidepressants side effects and is commonly prescribed in the USA; It has effects on norepinephrine and serotonin; see Tricyclics, Amitriptyline, and Pamelor;

Eldepryl (is selegine in pill form)—Eldepryl is an MAOI antidepressant. It is useful in neurology (for Parkinsonism) and in psychiatry (for Depression). At low doses, Eldepryl does not require a special diet, but at higher doses, it does require a special diet, which is complicated. It is usually used in higher doses when treating Depression. If a Depressed patient is taking a higher oral dose, then he will have two choices: either learn to follow the diet; or, use the Emsam patch which is absorbed directly through the skin and thus does not require a special diet. See MAOI;

Emsam (is a selegiline skin patch—see Eldepryl); patients taking Emsam need not follow dietary restrictions but still need to avoid certain drugs; see MAOI;

Escitalopram—see Lexapro

Etrafon—see Triavil

Fluoxetine—see Prozac

Fluvoxamine—see Luvox

GENERIC MEDICATIONS—these are supposed to be exact copies of the formula for the original branded medication: the chemical nature of the generic medication is FDA-guaranteed to be the same as branded, but the generic might be produced by different methods and processes; see BRANDED MEDICATIONS;

Ilex—see milnacipran

Imipramine—see Tofranil

Ionamin—is an amphetamine derivative primarily used as a diet pill. It is effective for weight control, but only while it is being taken continuously. Once the pill is stopped, the person is likely to regain weight unless she has made major modifications to her lifestyle in the meantime: daily aerobics, non-caloric beverages, low-fat diet incorporating protein of high biological value, and so on. It has occasionally been used in Depression as a secondary drug. Like all the amphetamines, it can have long-term effects on the heart and blood vessels.

Isocarboxazid—see Marplan

Lexapro—is an SSRI which is the "purified" form of Celexa

Ludiomil—is a medication similar to the tricyclics, but having a unique structure that seems to give it slightly different side effects as well as somewhat different therapeutic effects. When it was first marketed in the USA, its competitors created the impression that it causes seizures—that risk is minimal but can increase if very high doses are used. In reality, most antidepressants have been reported to cause rare seizures if used at high doses, Anafranil and Wellbutrin, for example. Any possible risk of seizure can be minimized by starting Ludiomil at a low dose and increasing slowly—which is really how all psychoactive medications should be prescribed, anyway. Ludiomil can be used for anxious depression, dysthymia, or Depression. It has a well-rounded spectrum of beneficial effects and side effects: not overly stimulating or sedating and does not usually cause significant weight gain. It favors activation of the nor-epinephrine system, and hence, can be used—if necessary— with low dose serotonin antidepressants (SSRI's, such as Lexapro or Prozac) to produce a broader range of antidepressant activity. Low-dose Ludiomil (generic name maprotiline) is used extensively in Europe and Latin America in the ways that we use Elavil and Doxepin. See Tricyclics;

Luvox—is another of the SSRI antidepressants. It has good antidepressant effects and is used to treat Depression in Europe. Apart from its antidepressant effects, it also exerts very powerful anti-obsessive properties—more powerful than any of the other SSRI's. All of the SSRI's have some degree of anti-obsessive properties, but Luvox has it in abundance. Its parent drug company decided to bring it to market here as a treatment for obsessive-compulsive disorders, with its only competition at that time, having been Nardil (an MAOI) and Anafranil (a Tricyclic); hence, each of the three medications carved out its own niche (for the treatment of obsessions and compulsions). American psychiatrists already knew that Luvox was a potent antidepressant and did not hesitate to use it in Depressions that had been resistant to many other medications, and in these cases it often worked well. The big drawback of Luvox is that it greatly interferes with many other medications. For this reason, it is not ideal for elderly patients or anyone who is taking a lot of other medicines—its target audience consists of compulsive young and middle-aged men and women.

MAOI—is a family of antidepressants that are very effective for certain types of Depressions; they have a number of side effects such as stimulation, insomnia, flushing, changes in blood pressure, sexual problems; a person taking these drugs must follow the MAOI diet; these drugs should be prescribed only by a psychiatrist because they can be very dangerous and require a significant amount of medical oversight; MAOI's can have fatal interactions when mixed with a number of other prescription medications, OTC medications, and certain foods; the MAOI antidepressants are Nardil, Parnate, Selegiline, Emsam, and Marplan; Eutonyl is no longer used; Emsam does not normally require following the special diet but does forbid a number of prescription medications; newer European MAOI's are safer, but the drug companies are certain that there is no profit from bringing these medications to America (the target market is too small and the medications are not as "user-friendly" as the already established SSRI and SSNRI antidepressants);

Maprotiline—see Ludiomil

Marplan—is one of the old MAOI medications and has a very tiny following. It should be *prescribed only by psychiatrists* who are familiar with its effects and complicated side effects.

MEDICATION—refers to prescription medicines (R_x medicines)

Milnacipran—is a French antidepressant, which has been available overseas since 1996; it is now FDA-approved to treat fibromyalgia in the USA (and it could be used "off-label" for Depression).

Mirtazapine—see Remeron

Nardil—this is an old MAOI antidepressant. It *should be prescribed only by psychiatrists* who are familiar with its complex suite of side effects and beneficial effects. It is very helpful for select patients. It is hard to believe now, but Nardil was once a novel antidepressant with a popular following. It debuted at a time when there were only three families of antidepressants: stimulants/amphetamines, MAOI, and a few Tricyclics. When Nardil was a big "hammer," it was used on many "nails." It has since then been superseded by many new classes of antidepressants, most of which are considerably safer. Nardil is still very effective for certain types of Depression, panic, obsessions, and "hysteroid dysphoria." A person taking Nardil needs to follow a very specific and restricted diet, otherwise she may run the risk of having a stroke or other cardiovascular misadventure. When it is prescribed in the usual method, it will not have any effects until between the fifth and sixth weeks of treatment. These patients need to have regular monitoring of blood pressure and pulse. Side effects can often include flushing, dizziness, sexual problems, and insomnia.

Nefazodone—see Serzone

Norpramin—this is the branded name of Desipramine, a Tricyclic that is the "purified" form of Tofranil (Imipramine) and as such it has milder side effects, compared to the other tricyclics. It favors the norepinephrine system and can be used carefully with low doses of SSRI's, if need be.

Nortriptyline—see Pamelor

OTC—these are all the medications sold Over The Counter (without a prescription)—some of these can cause death if mixed with MAOI's; some OTC's can cause confusion and urine retention in the elderly;

Pamelor—this is the branded name of the Tricyclic, nortriptyline, the "purified" form of Elavil; its popularity is waning somewhat. It has effects on serotonin and norepinephrine. See Elavil

Parnate—is an MAOI antidepressant that requires a special diet, the MAOI diet. Parnate actually has an amphetamine structure, but it is not addicting like the amphetamines. Parnate is the most stimulating MAOI.

Paroxetine—see Paxil

Paxil—is similar to the other SSRI drugs with a few exceptions. Paxil can have histamine-like effects, causing hunger and, thus, weight gain. At very high doses, it may demonstrate mild stimulation due to a slight norepinephrine-like effect that might appear in some patients. Paxil is probably the likeliest of the SSRI medications to cause "discontinuation syndrome." Paxil is also very effective for premature ejaculation (see SSRI); its generic name is paroxetine: Paxil is the HCl (hydrochloro) version and Pexeva is the mesylate (methane-sulfonate) version;

Phenelzine—see Nardil

Pristiq—is the "purified" form of Effexor and usually requires no dosage adjustments, it is thus quite "user-friendly" in this regard—see Effexor.

Protriptyline—see Vivactil

Prozac—Prozac appeared in the 1980's and was the first of a new group of antidepressants, which came to be called the SSRI's. Its basic chemical structure is similar to that of amphetamines, yet it is not addicting. When it first appeared, it was quickly recognized as a vast advance in the treatment of Depression because it is a strong activator of the brain hormone serotonin; it can be activating (in some cases too much so); and, it is safe in overdose (very important property in any antidepressant). As time went on, we also learned to mix it with other antidepressants for enhanced anti-Depression activity. As far as its activating properties, it—like most antidepressants—should not be prescribed to manic or psychotic patients who are exquisitely sensitive to antidepressants' activating properties. In these types of patients, antidepressants can set off a manic episode or a psychotic rage, which can be a very harrowing experience for the patient and those in his surroundings. Prozac received a bad [undeservedly] reputation from which it has never recovered, in the sense that I still see first-time patients who refuse even to try Prozac. It can be used in Depression, Bulimia, and obsessions. It is approved for use in children and teenagers. It can cause rash. See also SSRI's.

Psychostimulants—see Stimulants

Remeron—is a sedating antidepressant which can be given in the evening to promote sleep for the night, and its residual effects provide antidepressant effects on the following day. It is also quite agreeable for use in recovering alcoholics. Remeron can cause hunger and fluid retention—and hence, weight gain. (It is the "purified" form of an even more sedating European antidepressant, mianserin); A number of patients do not like its sedation or other side effects. For those who tolerate it well, it is very helpful. If experiencing weird dreams from bedtime dosing, then take Remeron much earlier in the evening instead of at bedtime. It is not likely to cause significant sexual side-effects; it is available in a special "Sol-tab" tablet that dissolves on the tongue, quite effective for patients who can not or will not swallow.

Ritalin—see Stimulant antidepressants

RLS—see Restless Legs Syndrome in the Vocabulary at the end of the book

Savella—see milnacipran

Selegiline—see Eldepryl, Emsam, and MAOI;

Sertraline—see Zoloft

Serzone (no longer routinely used in USA, but still available); it is a mild antidepressant without sexual side effects; long-term use of Serzone carries a very slight risk of liver failure (about one-two in a million); patients who have been taking it for many years need to be educated about this risk and are encouraged to switch to different medications; the few rare patients who do well only on Serzone and refuse to change, need to have blood testing of liver function every two-three months, although this measure probably does not offer much protection or forewarning; I have limited use of this drug to patients with end-stage kidney failure and for those who have taken it for a long time.

Sinequan—is the branded name for Doxepin. Sinequan is a very popular Tricyclic antidepressant. It is almost as popular as Elavil. (In Europe and Latin America, Ludiomil would typically be used in low doses in the way that Elavil and Sinequan are used in America.)

Doxepin has effects on the "brain hormones," serotonin and norepinephrine. It can cause sedation, weight gain, deep sleep, low blood pressure (dizziness), and drying effects (ideal for hay fever/ sinus sufferers); however, excess drying effects can result in blurred vision, prostate problems, urine retention, constipation, and dry mouth. It also has anti-acid properties and was used decades ago as a stomach pill for ulcer patients. The weight gain can aggravate diabetes (by causing further weight gain) and arthritis (by creating more weight to be dragged around); abdominal weight gain can aggravate the labor of breathing in emphysema. Doxepin can control itching in certain skin conditions. In low dosage, it can be ideal for anxious young (alcoholic) men or for patients who want to dry out some part of their organ system. It lasts a long time in the body and has some interactions with regular medical drugs (excess sedation), especially with other sedating medications and blood pressure pills. For all these reasons, it should usually be avoided in elderly patients. It is available as a liquid. Blood levels are available, too, as a guide to dosing.

SNRI—these antidepressants have effects on the norepinephrine system of feel-good "brain hormones"; Strattera (Atomoxetine) is a European SNRI antidepressant available in America; it is marketed here for ADHD. Vestra (reboxitene) is another European SNRI antidepressant; Savella (milnacipran) has notable SNRI activity.

SSNRI—these drugs have effects on both the serotonin and norepinephrine system, hence they function as SSRI + SNRI. SSNRI's available in the USA today are Cymbalta, Effexor, Pristiq, and Savella: these drugs have varying effects on serotonin and norepinephrine, depending upon: (1) which drug is taken; (2) the person's genetic ability to use the drug; and (3) the dosage range. The Tricyclics, such as Elavil, also have this type of dual action, but the Tricyclics also have a suite of effects on other bio-chemical systems of the body; see SSRI, also;

SSRI—this is a group of medications with effects on the serotonin system of feel-good "brain hormones" and includes Celexa, Lexapro, Luvox, Paxil, Prozac, and Zoloft. As a group they have a number of similar properties and side effects. These medications are effective in a large number of Depressed patients and are also effective in many types of Depression, such as Major Depression, Minor Depression, Dysthymia, as well as being effective in a number of Anxiety disorders and Obsessive-Compulsions (not covered in this book); additionally, they may control premature ejaculation (Paxil). SSRI Side effects can include dizziness, nausea, diarrhea, headache, confusion, nervousness, sedation, as well as rash and bruising. If a rash appears, the medication should be stopped immediately; a less serious side effect is bruising that is related to serotonin receptors on our platelets; the other side effects are typical of the first week of treatment, and patients should be encouraged to continue the SSRI—this is the reason why I usually start patients with a half dose in the first week: less discomfort. One of the more distressing side effects is that of the so-called "Discontinuation Syndrome," which represents a group of symptoms that may occur in patients who suddenly quit taking an SSRI (or SSNRI). This occurs in only a fraction of patients, usually those who have adapted well to the drug and like its positive effects but have decided to quit it—for one reason or another. The patients who did not like the SSRI usually do not have this reaction because it either did not help them or caused a lot of annoying physical side effects (and their bodies are probably glad to be rid of it). The Discontinuation symptoms will appear within a day or two (three-four days with Prozac) and will last for a few-several days. The symptoms are usually those of "flu", such as aches, headaches, dizziness, as well as racing thoughts or lethargy. This is technically not withdrawal. Withdrawal is a term we use for the possibly life-threatening symptoms and signs that drug addicts or alcoholics experience if they do not get their regular dose of addicting drug or alcohol; symptoms of withdrawal are vastly more disabling that those of Discontinuation, which produces no [direct] lethal effects. It is entirely reasonable to give a Discontinuation patient time off from work during this reaction, as if he had the "flu." If a second SSRI is being chosen as a replacement for the first SSRI, the switch can often be done expeditiously over a long weekend without too much discomfort (but there may be some symptoms of adjustment for a few days). The successful outcome of this maneuver depends upon the half-life of the first SSRI, the patient's reaction, and the psychiatrist's philosophy/experience.

Stimulant Antidepressants—are also called Psychostimulants, which should give you a good idea of their effects and potency; in a sense, any antidepressant that causes euphoria could be a psycho-stimulant, but it is generally accepted that this term refers specifically to the amphetamines, Ritalin, Cylert, and several other types of medications, all of which are habit-forming/addictive;

Strattera—is a European antidepressant used for ADDH in the USA; it has a modest antidepressant effect; it can cause nausea, dizziness, buzziness; men are prone to an odd sexual sensation from Strattera, which is like a cremasteric reflex, a sensation of testicles being pulled up into the pelvis;

Surmontil—is a Tricyclic antidepressant with short-acting properties; it is like Sinequan but with all the side effects much reduced; it may help onset of sleep;

Tofranil—is a Tricyclic antidepressant with all around generalized side effects and with a number of uses: most importantly, it is an effective antidepressant which tends to be sedating in lower doses, but more activating in much higher doses; it can be used in obsessive compulsions and panic-anxiety—it worked fairly well when it was about the only prescription we had for these purposes; it could be used in ADHD but its use in teenage boys has been possibly loosely associated with two or three sudden heart attacks per year in this country; its "purified" form is called Norpramin (Desipramine); see the story of Bartholomew;

Tranylcypromine—see Parnate

Trazodone—this is the generic name for Desyrel, a popular medication;

Triavil—is a fixed combination of Elavil and Perphenazine and seems to work better than taking each drug in two separate pills; it was used in psychotic Depressions, involutional melancholy, and Depression linked to chronic pain; also marketed as Etrafon;

Tricyclic antidepressants—the members of this chemical family are all similar in function and share certain side effects: mild sedation, dry mouth, blurred vision, constipation, urine retention, dry skin, changes in blood pressure and pulse, or vivid dreams. Any of these side effects is possible, but most people only have one or two of the side effects, most of which can be improved by various maneuvers, such as changing the dosing or by using "side effect" drugs. Stimulating Tricyclics (Vivactil, Norpramin) should not be taken at bedtime as they will cause "weird" or vivid dreams—these medications should be taken during the daytime; even some of the traditionally sedating Tricyclics may disrupt sleep and so they should be taken earlier in the evening. Some tricyclics may cause a rash (Vivactil, notably), whereas Sinequan can be used to decrease itching (due to its antihistamine properties, not its antidepressant properties); these medications can be helpful for certain kinds of chronic pain (shingles, back pain, other pains); these medications may increase appetite (not Vivactil), but unfortunately will not help anorexia; Vivactil can cause some cardiovascular side effects and should not be used in the elderly; Doxepin can cause low blood pressure and likewise should be avoided in the elderly.

Trimipramine—see Surmontil

Venlafaxine—see Effexor (and its "purified" version, Pristiq)

Vivactil—is an activating Tricyclic which I use a lot as a second or third tier medication in Depressed women; it is especially helpful if these women report extreme stimulation from SSRI's, Effexor, or Wellbutrin. It can have cardiac effects and prospective patients need a baseline EKG (heart wave test); Vivactil can be used in ADHD; when used in combination with Effexor, the mixture is referred to as "California Rocket Fuel"; it is not ideal for use in the elderly;

Wellbutrin—can be stimulating to some people due to the fact that it can activate levels of two major stimulating antidepressant "brain hormones" (dopamine and norepinephrine). Its stimulating side effects are most apparent in the first one to three weeks of treatment (especially in the first week). This is one reason that it is not usually considered a first-line medication for agitated Depression, Psychotic Depression, or in any Depression that could not tolerate stimulation (such as patients who are already over-stimulated from asthma medicines, prednisone, or who have a family history of bipolar depression, and other clinical situations). Alcoholics and drug addicts in early recovery may also find that these stimulant effects disrupt their serenity which in turn could lead to a disruption of sobriety. Furthermore, Wellbutrin may cause seizures and should not be given to patients with epilepsy or bulimia. Alcoholics in early recovery may also be at higher risk of seizures. When I start patients on Wellbutrin, the experience is much more tolerable when starting with very small doses and then increasing up to normal adult doses over the next few weeks—this maneuver is also thought to reduce the risk of any epileptic seizure. Wellbutrin's main side effects are constipation, dizziness, and sensations of "head buzzing" or ringing ears. Since it is derived from the old diet pill, Tenuate, it is rarely associated with significant weight gain. Wellbutrin and Serzone are the two antidepressants least likely to cause undesirable sexual side effects. Oftentimes, patients may report that they felt stimulated in the first week of treatment, but then start to feel calmer after three weeks: they like this effect and it seems to parallel what happens when we use antidepressant medication to treat ADHD (All the treatments for ADHD are simply antidepressants of various classes). Wellbutrin has an added convenience of being available in short-acting pills, intermediate-acting pills, and long-lasting pills. Some people who like Wellbutrin's mild stimulation derive great benefit from it in the daytime, but then complain of insomnia (at bedtime). These people can be given short-acting Wellbutrin that should wear off by nighttime.

Zoloft—is an SSRI drug with a generally well-rounded side effect profile and is useful for various kinds of Depression and many Anxiety Disorders. It is very effective in low doses for geriatric Depression: See SSRI's.

Secondary Medications
and Mood Stabilizers

Apart from the main antidepressant, there are three more categories of medications that can be added to the primary antidepressant. These medications are useful—and often necessary—in the treatment of severe Depressions. These categories are: secondary medications, mood stabilizers, and side effect pills. The secondary medications include

Abilify, Risperdal, Zyprexa, Buspar, Trazodone, and others. The mood stabilizers can be used in Cycling Depressions: Depakote, Lamictal, Lithium, Tegretol, Trileptal, and others. For more information regarding the three categories of "add-on" medications (including side effect pills) for the treatment of Depression, see my second book, *Defeating Depression.*

Discontinuation Syndrome
See under SSRI's in the list above

SIDE EFFECTS COMMON TO MOST ANTIDEPRESSANT MEDICATIONS

Antidepressants can have different side effects depending upon their chemical classification. Here are a few generalizations about the most common side effects of most antidepressants:

AGE—elderly people need less of any medication, sometimes half the usual adult dosage. The very elderly may need only one-third or one-fourth dosage. In general, the elderly should avoid medications that cause confusion, such as Tricyclics; similar caution should be used also if prescribing them Remeron and Paxil. Effexor can worsen their blood pressure sometimes. Prozac has a very long half-life and is not a first choice treatment; Luvox should definitely be avoided in the elderly as it interacts with so many of their regular medical medications. MAOI medications are too complicated and dangerous. Stimulants can, however, be used as a primary antidepressant or as a secondary medication in small doses (such as 5 mg of Ritalin). Most medications should be reduced in old age—not just psychiatric medications, but many medications.

ANXIETY/RESTLESSNESS/AGITATION—this may occur in the first week of treatment with SSRI, SSNRI, and Wellbutrin. This side effect usually disappears. One treatment strategy is to start with only a fraction of the usual dosage for the first weeks. If this side effect occurs in later treatment phases, there may be numerous factors involved, depending upon the individual case.

GENDER—there is usually no need to alter the doses based on gender; in other words, men do not necessarily need a higher dose of medication than do women. The only exception may be that of petite frail very elderly women who may need only one-fourth the usual adult dose, whereas very elderly men may need one-third dose.

HEADACHES—can be common at certain phases of treatment, but should not last long. If headaches become a problem, there are various maneuvers available depending on the medication involved and all the details of the case. The cause of the headache must be determined. If related to elevated blood pressure, the medication may need to be changed or the blood pressure, controlled. If due to an interaction with another medication, then other steps will need to be taken. If the headache is caused by the antidepressant medication, then the mechanism of cause needs to be understood and managed. It is not possible to give a general statement about treating headaches, since there are multiple causes and types of headaches: treatment is often on a very individualized basis. In about half the cases, the headache can be managed and removed, and in another fraction of cases, the Depression treatment may need to be changed.

MENTAL—any of the medications may variously cause sleepiness, mild confusion, impaired concentration, racing thoughts, insomnia, or alertness during the first weeks of treatment. These effects usually normalize by the third or fourth week of treatment after which the patient feels much better as he will often experience a pleasant combination of alertness, improved concentration, prolonged attention span, inner peacefulness and contentment, and mood stability without restlessness or hyperactivity.

RASH: can be caused by Lamictal, Vivactil, and any of the SSRI's or SSNRI's (in truth, any synthetic medication can cause rash); any **rash caused by Lamictal** can be dangerous and even **fatal**. If Lamictal causes a rash, stop the medication immediately and go to the ER (hospital). If any of the other antidepressants cause a rash, stop the medication and get in touch with your prescriber. The most serious allergic reactions often occur within a week of starting a new medication. If the person continues the antidepressant in the presence of a rash, she could have a very serious reaction requiring a trip to the nearest ER. If any medication rash is accompanied by gasping and blue skin, this is an extreme emergency that requires instantaneous treatment. Once a person has had an allergic reaction to an antidepressant, then that drug should never be taken again. If that drug is in a large family of drugs, some of the others in that chemical family may not be safe, either (Tricyclics for example)—this does not necessarily apply to the SSRI's and SNRI's because none of these are really in the same chemical family.

If a rash occurs after months of treatment, then the situation may not be so dire. There may be an intervening factor that is triggering the rash. The intervening factor may be the introduction of a new pill, vitamin, exotic food, soap, or any substance that contains chemical dyes; FD&C approved dyes are numerous and found in many drugs, cosmetics, and foodstuff. A search should be instigated to ferret out the aggravating cause. If it can be identified, then it should be eliminated and the antidepressant resumed at tiny doses. At any rate, a late-appearing rash should prompt the patient to stop the medicine until the doctor(s) can identify a cause or reason for the appearance of the rash. Late-occurring rashes might have dermatological causes. A visit to a dermatologist for a second opinion may be helpful—see Ida's story. (For a complete list of side effects, see Table 7 in Section V in my book *Defeating Depression*.)

SEIZURES—many antidepressant medications are listed as possibly causing seizures, but that occurs rarely in real-life practice unless patients start with too high a dose—or take an excess amount of medication in an attempt to feel better faster. The seizure rates may be quoted as high as 2% for some antidepressants; those studies were probably done using normal or high-normal doses, and some of the volunteers for those drug studies might not have been carefully screened.

SEX—many of these medications have undesirable effects on sexual performance, specifically effects of delaying or even preventing orgasm (men and women). Wellbutrin and Serzone (and Buspar) do not affect sexual function. Trazodone can very rarely cause *priapism* in men (prolonged painful erections which can become a medical-surgical emergency); otherwise, Trazodone is "sex-neutral" (it has no real positive or negative sexual side effects). Few of the antidepressants cause outright impotence—unlike antipsychotics and blood pressure pills that can cause temporary impotence. All of these above sexual side effects disappear once the antidepressant medication is stopped (except for emergency treatment of *priapism* which can result in permanent impotence—see Desyrel in the list above). Remeron seems to be sex-neutral, also.

SLEEP/SLEEPINESS—in the first couple weeks, any medication can cause excess sleep, disrupted sleep, daytime drowsiness, or loss of sleep (insomnia). If these symptoms do not improve after a week or two, the doctor may need to make certain adjustments. Some medications (Tricyclics) may be very helpful for sleep, but then a few months into treatment, they may cause vivid dreams or arousals in the wee hours. These symptoms can often be eliminated by dosing the medication earlier in the day or in the afternoon before bedtime. This is also true of Effexor. SSRI's may shorten the sleep cycle, and there are several adjustments that can be made, commonly adding Trazodone at bedtime (women) or for men, adding bed-time doses of Vistaril, Remeron, Neurontin, Buspar, L-Tryptophan, Doxepin, and so on.

SWELLING / INCREASE in FLUID WEIGHT: this happens notably in women taking Remeron (swollen ankles); less commonly, with Trazodone.

TREMBLING/SHAKINESS—this may occur if the blood level is too high.

WEIGHT—most antidepressants cause weight gain, sometimes modest and sometimes only a few vanity pounds. But, some antidepressants can cause considerable weight gain. Weight gain is especially pronounced with Remeron, Paxil, and Sinequan (and other Tricyclic antidepressants). Weight gain is modest with Ludiomil and Norpramin. Weight gain should be low to minimal with most SSRI's, SNRI's, SSNRI's, and Trazodone; very low weight gain to none, is usually characteristic of treatment with Vivactil, Serzone, and Wellbutrin.

Among the secondary medications and mood stabilizers, spectacular weight gain may occur with Zyprexa and Seroquel. Moderate weight gain may occur with Lithium, whereas Depakote usually causes less weight gain. Lamictal, Tegretol, Trileptal, and Abilify have little effect on weight; Buspar has none.

BLACK BOX WARNINGS

Black Box is a warning that the FDA (Food and Drug Administration) assigns to medications that might have lethal side effects (causing death). Most recently, the FDA has issued a Black Box warning for any and all antidepressants used in young adults under age twenty-five. The Black Box warning in these cases is an alert that the medications could lead to suicidal tendencies in Depressed children, teenagers, and young adult patients. This whole hullabaloo started a few years ago when a couple SSRI's were supposedly linked to teenage suicides. Soon thereafter, all the SSRI antidepressants came under attack amidst claims that they "cause suicide" in children and teenagers; the SSRI's are Celexa, Lexapro, Luvox, Paxil, Prozac, and Zoloft. The FDA wished to give the impression of being appropriately responsive to this issue, so they put black box warnings on any SSRI antidepressant used in children and teens. Later the FDA expanded the Black Box warning to include anyone under age twenty-five using SSRI's. Later still, this warning mushroomed into a general declaration that *all* antidepressants (not just SSRI's) "could cause suicide" in anyone under the age of twenty-five. This created a lot of hubbub in the news and among psychiatrists, as one can well imagine. Some of the Black Box warnings look scary and can be very lengthy. The warning for SSRI's is short.

This is the Black Box warning for the SSRI's:

> ANTIDEPRESSANTS INCREASED THE RISK OF SUICIDAL THINKING
> AND BEHAVIOR (SUICIDALITY) IN SHORT-TERM STUDIES IN CHILDREN
> AND ADOLESCENTS WITH MAJOR DEPRESSION...ANYONE CONSIDERING
> THE USE OF [NAME OF DRUG] IN A CHILD OR ADOLESCENT MUST
> BALANCE THIS RISK FOR THE CLINICAL NEED. PATIENTS WHO ARE
> STARTED ON THERAPY SHOULD BE OBSERVED CLOSELY FOR CLINICAL
> WORSENING, SUICIDALITY, OR UNUSUAL CHANGES IN BEHAVIOR.
> FAMILIES AND CAREGIVERS SHOULD BE ADVISED OF THE NEED FOR
> CLOSE OBSERVATION AND COMMUNICATION WITH THE PRESCRIBER.

Most psychiatrists think that this black box warning for the SSRI antidepressants is absurd for the following reasons:

- Depression causes suicide (not the antidepressants that fight Depression)—suicide is an inherent risk in treating all Depressions.
- The larger the number of untreated cases of Depression in a population, then the larger the number of suicides: Depression predictably leads to suicide. The more severe the Depression, the higher the rates of suicide in untreated cases.
- Suicide rates have decreased due to the availability of modern antidepressants.
- Suicide is the third commonest cause of death in teenage boys and young men, regardless of any other variables, and has been so, even before we started blithely and routinely drugging our children/teenagers.

And if we would like to continue picking apart this SSRI black box warning, consider this:

- The [few] studies were short-term, not long-term.
- Any reasonable doctor and responsible parents would observe closely for "unusual changes in behavior," anyway. And finally,
- What constitutes "unusual changes in behavior" in teenagers?

This serves as a further reminder that antidepressants are synthetic chemicals made in a factory (except the earth salt, Lithium) and should be treated as medicinal in low doses and poisonous in higher doses. It is entirely possible that certain toxic effects occur when blood levels of these antidepressants rise too high. Since most of these medications have no routinely available blood levels (yet), we do not know precisely. The best place to start is with advocating for routine availability of blood levels of SSRI's and all antidepressants—this might be the best way to monitor treatment with these drugs instead of looking out for "unusual" teenage behaviors.

Apart from that, here is a list of all the antidepressants that carry Black Box warnings for all patients of all ages based on fatal chemical reactions of the medication (the serious side effects are inside parentheses after the name of the medication):

- Antidepressant Serzone (liver failure requiring liver transplant)
- Antidepressant Stimulants (addiction and heart damage): these antidepressant medications are amphetamines, Cylert, and Ritalin (which are also used to treat ADHD)
- Antidepressant SSRI's (suicidal behaviors in young people and children): Celexa, Lexapro, (Luvox), Paxil, Prozac, Zoloft
- Antidepressants in general (suicidal behaviors in young people?)
- MAOI antidepressants (stroke)

This is a scary-looking list. But there is a much longer list that includes many other psychiatric medications (see Section XII in my book *Defeating Depression*). This is why patients should really see a psychiatrist for psychiatric treatment instead of getting "curbside consults" with their primary doctor. I do not prescribe medical medications for diabetes, blood pressure, asthma, etc to my patients, and I would certainly never prescribe such drugs if they were black-boxed; hence, I question the wisdom of having non-psychiatrists prescribing black-box psychiatric medications. Given the new black-box status of antidepressants, I find the promiscuous prescribing of these drugs by non-psychiatrists to be quite curious.

PREGNANCY

Some women are taking antidepressants for relatively mild forms of Depression. Some of these mild Depressions do not absolutely need to be medicated during pregnancy—except for smoking cessation, which is important for fetal well-being. At the other extreme, women with severe Depression may require major medications in pregnancy. However, some of these types of medications can expose the baby to risks of serious malformations, which will likely last for its lifetime. These malformations can be visible (physical deformities) or invisible (lifelong behavioral or emotional problems). The medicines might even result in premature delivery or stillbirth. The best starting place is to arrange psychiatric disorders according to their severity, that is, whether they are mild, moderate, or severe:

- Mild disorders would include Reactive Depression, minor Depression, Winter Depression, (mild) Dysthymia and Anxious Depression
- Moderate disorders would include Major Depression, (moderate) Dysthymia, and agitated Depression
- Severe disorders are Manic-Depression, Bipolar Depression, Psychotic Depression, and Severe Major Depressions
- Secondary Depressions should be treated by dealing with the primary cause of the Secondary Depression
- Winter Depression can be treated with artificial or natural sunlight which is not known to harm babies

Women with mild disorders should fare well unmedicated during pregnancy. These mild cases might choose to do weekly therapy with a therapist. This serves two purposes: first, therapy alone can provide a sense of well-being; second, the therapist can track a pregnant patient's general mood status, and if the patient is slipping from a mild to a moderate Depression, then the patient can be directed immediately to the therapist's supervising psychiatrist. Women with moderate and severe cases are advised to discuss treatment options with both the obstetrician and the psychiatrist (also, hopefully, with the father of the baby). If a woman with moderate or severe Depression has been receiving her psychoactive medicines from her family doctor, then she might consider consulting a psychiatrist.

In order to help doctors and the public to wrestle with the thorny issue of psychiatric drugs in pregnancy, the FDA has devised an ABCDX rating system for drugs in pregnancy: the "A" list drugs are known to be safe in pregnancy. "D" drugs are quite risky. "X" drugs are very toxic in pregnancy and should be avoided at all costs. "B" and "C" drugs are intermediate between safe "A" drugs and the "D" or "X" drugs. However, it should not be inferred that all the drugs on the "B" list are completely safe; some of them are not necessarily known to be "good" in pregnancy—so far, they are just not known to be "bad." The letter grades should not be misconstrued to coincide exactly with medication quality and safety—but it may be. Some of these drugs on the "B" and "C" lists have not been completely "vetted" for use in pregnancy. In other words, there are not enough data to make a final decision. It is possible that some of these "B" and "C" lists might be re-assigned in the future. Paxil is a good example of a previously "C" listed drug that was downgraded to "D". For another example, Clozaril is a very toxic antipsychotic medication that is on the "B" list: this is probably not testimony that it is safe, but rather that there is too little experience using it in pregnancy.

Drugs on the "A' list are known to be safe in pregnancy (but no psychiatric medicine is on the "A" list). Drugs currently on the "B" or "C" list may have made those lists due to lack of negative data rather than due to proof of safety in pregnancy (or they may actually be known to be safe). We do know that "D" and "X" list drugs are not safe. Try to avoid "D" drugs during pregnancy and do definitely avoid "X" listed drugs during pregnancy.

Special cases: Buspar is a non-addicting anti-anxiety drug originally developed as an antidepressant (same family as Serzone and Trazodone) and retains some mild mood enhancement properties in some patients. Tegretol is more toxic in the first trimester than in the second and third trimesters.

<u>Antidepressants on the "A" list</u>: NONE

Antidepressants on the "B" list: *Cylert, Ludiomil* (and Buspar)

Antidepressants on the "C" list: include most antidepressants:
MAOI's: *(Nardil, Marplan, Parnate, Eldepryl)*
Mood Stabilizers: *Tegretol (2ⁿᵈ & 3ʳᵈ trimesters), Trileptal, Lamictal*
SSRI: *Prozac, Zoloft, Celexa, Lexapro, Luvox*
SSNRI/SNRI: *Cymbalta, Effexor, Pristiq, Strattera*
Stimulants: *Ritalin, Dexedrine, Provigil, Ionamin, Wellbutrin*
Triazolo-piperazines: *Trazodone and Serzone*
Tricyclics: *Asendin, Doxepin, Desipramine*
Secondary Medications: *Abilify, Zyprexa, Seroquel, Geodon, Risperdal, Loxitane,* Compazine

Antidepressants on the "D" list: Paxil and some Tricyclics:
SSRI: *Paxil*
Tricyclics: *Pamelor, Elavil, Triavil, Tofranil (Imipramine)*
Mood Stabilizers: *Lithium, Depakote, Tegretol (1ˢᵗ trimester)*
St. John's Wort?
Social Alcohol, Nicotine, (Aspirin)

Special Notes:
Tegretol is on the "D" list in the first trimester, but then on the "C" list in the second and third trimesters.

Antidepressants on the "X" list:
NONE but please note that alcoholic binge drinking is "X" (causing FAS, Fetal Alcohol Syndrome, with permanent brain damage)

General Guidelines:
- Paxil is an SSRI antidepressant drug that was recently demoted to "D" from "C." Some of the other SSRI drugs (Celexa, Lexapro, Luvox, Prozac, and Zoloft) are now being scrutinized. Some people who have gone back and run other statistical studies on Paxil believe that the "D" rating may not be totally deserved. Others predict that Zoloft also might be demoted to "D" list from the "C" list. There is a lot of anecdotal information on Prozac in pregnancy and it is not unfavorable.

- in Germany, the herb, St John's Wort, is treated as a prescription medicine because it is known to cause birth defects if used during pregnancy (it is also a very commonly used antidepressant in Germany; its Rx status there makes it cheaper in the pharmacy than if sold OTC). Nonetheless it is still sold in the USA without a prescription (buyer beware).
- Lithium can cause heart defects in babies.
- Some drugs for Bipolar condition cause major malformations: Depakote, Tegretol.
- Alcohol, cigarettes, and street drugs are all bad for the baby. Relatively heavy drinking during pregnancy can cause Fetal Alcohol Syndrome (FAS), which can result in permanent nervous defects and especially mental defects. Smoking affects the baby and should be avoided. Babies born to cocaine-addicted or heroin-addicted mothers go through drug withdrawal after they are born. (This is obviously a bad start for a new life.)
- herbs are dried plants that contain hundreds or thousands of chemicals. Beware! Unless you are familiar with all these chemicals, you should be cautious.
- Assume that all psychiatric drugs pass into the breast milk (and into the baby).
- It has been reported that SSRI antidepressants may delay the onset of lactation (milk-production) to three-four days post-partum. The significance of this factoid is unknown.

Some women who really need to be medicated during pregnancy should be aware of the level of safety or of danger that is inherent in their current medications. For this reason, the FDA has drawn up these general guidelines regarding drug safety during pregnancy. If you are ordering drugs from other countries, some of those countries also have their own safety rating systems that may resemble ours, but are not the same. If medication during pregnancy is essential, then you might want to "upgrade" your current medication. If you are currently taking a "D" or "X" rated drug, then at least you might have the chance to "upgrade" to a "B" or "C" rated drug during part or all of your pregnancy with the option to return to your usual medication after the baby is born. (For more information, see Chapter VI-4, *Everyone's Everyday Guide to Practical Psychiatry*)

V)-Therapeutics
Finding a Mental Health
Professional

Psychiatry is a new branch of Medicine, having started less than a century and a half ago. In such a short time, the practice has gone from "soft" neurology (treatment of hysteria) to abstract treatment philosophy with dream interpretation (Freud and psychoanalysis) to once-weekly one-hour therapy sessions (as shown in movies) to modern biological psychiatry (pills and lab tests). That is much more change than the rest of Medicine has experienced throughout the last few thousand years.

People who watch movies—especially old black and white movies—might be surprised on their first visit to a modern psychiatrist. They might expect to see a long leather couch and might expect a one-hour session, neither of which is likely if seeing a psychiatrist in the HMO system. There are still a few psychiatrists who practice in this manner, but they may also be in private practice and charge higher rates for this enhanced service. A patient can usually get what he needs today by going through the usual and customary modern practice system. If he is still not satisfied, then he could discuss this with his HMO or mental health professional. Apart from that, this chapter points out how to begin seeking treatment.

Your first appointment will probably be with one of four basic types of mental health professional: counselor, therapist, psychologist, or psychiatrist. The modern trend is to call them all "providers" (of clinical services). The differences among these providers are explained here.

Psychiatrists
A psychiatrist is an M.D. or D.O. who specializes in psychiatric medicine and its forms of treatment, such as prescribing medications and giving injections. Psychiatrists also order lab tests (blood tests) and talk to primary doctors about medical problems of their mutual patients. Psychiatric treatment typically includes initial interviews and short follow-up sessions as well as managing the prescription medications. *Psychoanalysts* are MD doctors who have received the classical Freudian training and analyze a patient's behaviors, speech, and dreams in great detail.

Psychologists
Psychologists hold a Ph.D. and clinical psychologists have a Psy.D. degree. They will typically see clients for once-weekly sessions of talk therapy. The Ph.D. has been trained to administer psychological testing, which is an extremely valuable service for clinical practice. Psychiatrists who would like a battery of psychological tests will typically send their patients to a psychologist for testing since psychiatrists are not trained to administer these types of tests. Anyone interested in finding a psychologist for talk therapy can start with either a Ph.D. or Psy.D.

Therapists
Therapists—also known as psychotherapists—typically hold a master's degree which permits them to do "talk therapy." Visits with a therapist usually cost less than sessions with a doctor of psychology.

Counselors likewise hold State certification.

GETTING STARTED:
The three commonest ways to find a provider are by word of mouth, by referral from the family doctor or by referral from the patient's health insurance plan. Occasionally patients may see ads in a publication or may choose somebody who is conveniently located nearby or has a convenient schedule, such as evening hours. The next step is to call the office and make an appointment. Prospective patients are allowed to ask about billing and fees over the telephone—or to ask about anything they wish—before coming in for the initial evaluation. Remember

that you are technically a potential "consumer" of psychiatric services. (Psychiatrists hate to have their patients referred to as "consumers," but some of the non-medical personnel do use this terminology.) As such, you are allowed to ask consumer-type questions. You should ask questions.

FIRST VISIT TO THE PROVIDER

Then comes the *initial visit* with the mental health provider at which time the patient can reach a preliminary opinion as to whether she wants to come back for a second appointment. If she definitely does not wish to come back, then she might state that she will call back after checking her schedule. Some undecided patients will make the second appointment in person but then call back later to cancel it. If a patient feels good about the first session, then she will probably make a second appointment and keep it. Some shy patients might make a second appointment with no intention of keeping it. When these patients do not show up for the second appointment, they will be billed. This behavior is usually a symptom of their underlying psychological distress or fear of asserting themselves.

It is perfectly legitimate for a new patient, such as Meg, to announce at the first session that she is in the process of seeking a provider, implying that she is assessing the provider to see if he is acceptable to her. She should pick someone with whom she feels comfortable and with whom she is able to communicate while articulating her feelings. It is also important for her to choose someone who is appropriate to her circumstances and with whom she can work on a long-term basis. She needs to find a provider with whom she feels engaged. If the first provider does not "click," then Meg should schedule an appointment with another provider.

On the first visit, the provider will typically make a diagnosis so that he can start treatment. In almost all cases (where the patient is willing to receive treatment), we want to start treatment immediately, because psychiatric illness is like a medical or surgical illness—left untreated, it will frequently get worse. Therefore, prompt treatment is important and relies upon a prompt, reasonable, and accurate diagnosis. Typically, all doctors will examine a new patient, whether we are psychiatric doctors, pediatricians, or surgeons. There are several steps to making a diagnosis:

1. We listen to Meg's story of how she came to feel Depressed—or if she does not think that she is Depressed—then we listen to what she thinks is ailing her;
2. If any family members have accompanied her, then they will give more objective background regarding how she came to feel and behave differently;
3. She will tell us what she is feeling (symptoms);
4. Then we will elicit (request information on) her medical history and ask for a list of all her current medications; we will inquire as to any drug or alcohol abuse;
5. We will ask about Depression and alcoholism in her family;
6. The doctor will exam her, which in psychiatry means looking at her and all the telltale signs that suggest that she is Depressed, signs such as soft voice, lack of enthusiasm, stooped shoulders, downcast gaze, crying, trembling, and so on
7. The doctor will then make a preliminary diagnosis.

Non-medical providers will not do such an examination, as they are interested only in the psychological issues.

Nowadays most insured Americans will be directed by their HMO to see a specific provider who has a contractual agreement with that HMO. The nature of these visits can be variable. In some cases, they may be very brief medication-oriented visits (ten to fifteen minutes) on an infrequent basis (every few weeks).

ONGOING THERAPY

This is the time (in weeks, months, years) that is spent in seeing a provider on a regular basis. The length of time in treatment will depend upon several factors. If a person has a persistent and serious Depression (such as a Cycling Depression), then the length of treatment may be for life. Patients with less serious problems may require shorter treatment times, maybe six months or a couple years. Some people may stay until they feel better, and then quit treatment until sometime in the future when they feel the need to return. Duration of treatment can be discussed in the first or second appointment. If the client feels comfortable with the therapist, then therapy will begin and continue until a future time when there will be a mutual decision to phase out therapy or decrease the frequency of visits.

Most psychiatrists will spend forty to sixty minutes on the first visit, although complex cases may require ninety minutes. However, follow-up appointments will be shorter, in the range of fifteen to thirty minutes (average of about twenty minutes) during which time the focus of the visit will be on medication dosages, side effects, lab tests, and the medical aspects of treatment.

If Meg starts with a psychiatrist but also needs therapy sessions with a psychologist, counselor, or therapist, then she will likely obtain a referral to see a provider who specializes in talk therapy and psychological issues. Conversely, if Meg starts with a therapist and needs medication then she will be referred to a psychiatrist. Therapists often focus on relationship problems. Counselors usually focus on one specific issue (drugs, alcohol), whereas psychologists may focus on more complex issues such as severe compulsive behaviors. A client with any serious legal problems might be well advised to start with a psychologist whose doctorate would carry more weight when dealing with third parties, such as lawyers.

Therapy should have a stated purpose (which issues to work out), a process and procedure, a goal, and a definable end-point after which the client should be more capable of functioning on her own. However, some people with horrific issues and a long history of abuses, like Tiffany, may need to feel consoled and supported in therapy for any number of years. Most clients do not require therapy of this duration or intensity. It is important that Tiffany and her provider try to formulate a reasonable treatment plan early on so that Tiffany might have a sense of how she is progressing in therapy and what her goals of success might be.

ENDING THERAPY

This refers to that time when a client like Tiffany would like to stop having regular appointments with the provider. She will eventually arrive at this point when therapy is not anticipated to provide much more benefit. This can be mutually decided and discussed. Usually the therapy will not be terminated abruptly, but will slowly be phased out and then there will come the last session. At this point, Tiffany will start to rely upon herself, being armed with what she has learned about herself in therapy. Therapy finally comes to an end as by mutual agreement. This is the time for Tiffany to try to "leave the nest and fly on her own." She will learn to use community resources and other sources of benefit and solace.

Some clients wish to end therapy prematurely, often due to financial constraints or changes of schedule. Clients such as Tiffany are free to leave the relationship whenever they choose to dismiss the provider, but it should be announced in advance in case the provider would wish to give cautionary feedback. In all cases, clients are always welcome to come back and continue therapy if there are too many unresolved issues.

PROVIDERS AND THE LAW

Doctor-patient relationship is essentially a legal contract that begins when the patient shows up for an appointment and when the doctor agrees to start treatment. The doctor agrees to give the patient "usual and customary" treatment and the patient agrees to pay the doctor for his services. These are mutual agreements. These same laws occur with psychologists, therapists, and counselors, also.

The provider has a *duty* to maintain *confidentiality* and not talk about the patient's case to people outside the doctor-patient relationship—this includes strangers as well as spouses and family members. Unless the patient had legally given the provider such permission. The rules of confidentiality are strict and must not be breached. As in all contractual situations, the patient—as well as the provider—also has obligations and privileges protected by ethics and laws.

Apart from this, the patient also has "privilege" (another legal term), which means that the patient can control or restrict any information released by the provider to third parties (this applies to situations in which the client requests that copies of her chart be sent to a third party). Sensitive information or information unrelated to the case can be subjected to patient privilege at the patient's request. This information is never released unless the patient requests that the information be released—often in cases where the patient is involved in a lawsuit and information is exchanged between the attorneys.

Absence of Confidentiality: there are exceptions to the Confidentiality rule in cases where a patient is actively homicidal or has confessed to murder. Another exception would include any legitimate reason to suspect child abuse (this also applies to elder abuse). All providers *must* report known or suspected child and elder abuse to the appropriate authorities.

SUMMARY

The whole treatment process can be somewhat complicated but only for a minority of patients. Most patients will have a very unremarkable experience. Anything that seems remarkable at first will have been—in hindsight—probably due to anxiety. This is how it works: You call your insurance company and they give you a list of mental health professionals. You call around and find someone who has openings. You make an appointment. You show up for intake (first appointment) and meet your prospective therapist/doctor. If you like that person, then you continue; otherwise, cancel the next appointment and start calling around all over again. If you are self-paying, try to find out who is good in your area, then call and make an appointment, etc.

And, when this whole talk therapy process is finished and you are able to have a mutual termination, then you are ready to make a "flight into health" to see how well you can "fly" on your own. If not well, then you can always come back to the "nest" for more therapy sessions.

Just remember that the mental health provider is licensed to deal with all these issues of concern, so you, the patient, must rely on trust to override fear at the earliest visits.

INTIMACY

It is illegal in all jurisdictions for any licensed health professional of any kind to go out on dates or sleep with his/her clients/patients. If this has happened to you, then you should notify the Licensing Board of the State where this happened. This would apply to all licensees: psychiatrists, psychotherapists, psychologists, and any other providers of medical/dental services.

PARTING THOUGHTS

All psychiatric diagnosis tends—to a certain degree—to be the doctor's opinion, so find a doctor whom you like and whose opinion you feel you can trust.

▶Remember: You can do a basic <u>background check on your provider</u> at the:

<u>State Medical Board website</u>
or on
<u>the National Practitioner Data Bank (NPDB) website</u>

~CONCLUSION~

From this book, you should be able to appreciate that diagnosis and treatment of Depression is best left to psychiatrists, and in some cases, Depression treatment can be a subspecialty of psychiatry. Some universities and hospitals have a special Mood Disorders Clinic within the department of psychiatry. Some people think that Depression is an all-or-nothing event, like an on-off switch. Either Meg is Depressed or not. Now you know that there are many faces, sources, causes, and forms of Depression. They exist along a continuum or spectrum and can all blend into each other. You can see now that:

- there are many types of Depression;
- each type of Depression can have different degrees of incapacity;
- each type of Depression can have various causes—or no known cause at all;
- two or more types of Depression may be present in the same person at the same time;
- there are other treatments available besides pills and synthetic chemicals;
- effective treatment depends upon sorting out all these above factors; and,
- more serious Depressions will require more complicated and in-depth treatment(s).

Euthymia refers to a feeling of well-being. Euthymia is the goal for which we strive in treatment of all Depressions. Sometimes it can be achieved by use of medications, sometimes we can approach it but never arrive, and in a few cases, it never happens: *"Is this as good as it gets?"* (Jack Nicholson asks in the movie of the same name; his character apparently had OCD and narcissism).

Public perception of Depression still continues to be negative. Depressives are sometimes trivialized as lazy and unmotivated. This is tragic because Depressives mostly want the same things as everyone else: happiness, family warmth, social acceptance, as well as nice cars, homes, and vacations—but it is out of reach because they have lost their earning potential—probably through no fault of their own. Depression is not a choice, it is an accident. It is a disease that visits itself upon its victims and mows them down. Chronically Depressed people are often judged as being what they are not. Yet they are not necessarily lazy, shiftless, unmotivated, sad, or irritable, but that the Depression makes them that way. The shock is not that Depressives have fallen so far. No, the miracle is that treated Depressives are still able to get up every day and eke through their existence. Those who are still working should be applauded for their "stick-to-it-ness" instead of being scorned. They have not chosen the easy way out (which would be that of applying for disability payments). I have observed even a wide spectrum of personal reactions from mental health professionals regarding this issue.

The only solution for Depressives is to get on the road to recovery and meet other people who are on that same road. Others who are on different roads may slowly [choose to] slip off onto the horizon...but that is beyond your control. Know what you can and cannot control and then choose wisely.

Good Luck and Be Well!

VOCABULARY OF TERMS, ABBREVIATIONS, AND DEFINITIONS

ADHD—Attention Deficit Hyperactivity Disorder is a disorder that appears before age seven; it shares symptoms with Depression such as decreased attention span and concentration as well as listlessness or restlessness; all the medications used for ADHD treatment are antidepressants, such as stimulant antidepressants (see below), as well as Strattera, Effexor, Wellbutrin, Tofranil, and others.

APA—American Psychiatric Association: publishes the DSM which is the official handbook used in America to diagnose (but not treat) psychiatric disorders.

"BRAIN HORMONE"—refers to the various bio-chemicals in the brain that regulate behavior and mood; since the middle of the XXth Century, we have developed a theory that Depression is related to deficits of one or more of these, the three most important of which are presumed to be dopamine, serotonin, and norepinephrine (properly called neurotransmitters); Any factor that lowers the brain levels of these bio-chemicals is thought to cause Depression, whereas medications and drugs that raise the levels of the three main "brain hormones" make people feel happy/non-Depressed, presumably; apart from these three main bio-chemicals, there are others present in smaller concentrations and new ones are still being identified and discovered.

BRAND-NAME MEDICATION, BRANDED MEDICATION, PATENT MEDICINES, TRADE-NAME MEDICATIONS— these four terms all refer to the same concept: the branded medication is the original medication which was invented by and first marketed by the parent drug company; this company has an exclusive right to make and sell its own creation until the patent expires. After the drug company's seventeen year patent expires, then generic versions of the branded drug are allowed to be sold; when very popular branded drugs become generic, there may be two or more generic companies marketing generic versions—if this is the case, some patients may notice a difference between the branded and generic drugs—and may also notice a difference between generic versions made by different generic drug companies; for this reason, it is wise to try to stabilize on one particular version and stick with it; unpopular branded drugs may not have any generic alternatives available—or the parent company may simply repackage its own branded drug in a different sized and colored pill and make a virtual monopoly of the branded and the [only] generic version (in this case, the generic will not be cheap); if the parent company continues to make only its branded version and if one generic drug company is the sole provider of the generic version, then the generic version will also not be cheap; In these latter cases, you might ask, 'so what's the big deal about an only generic version if it is still relatively pricey?'—the big deal is that your HMO will offer you the generic at a much cheaper rate (the same generic co-pay you pay for all your other generic drugs: the costly generic is only costly if you have no health insurance prescription plan). Examples: (1) when Prozac was under patent protection, Eli Lilly (d/b/a Dista Corp) had the exclusive right to manufacture and sell Prozac starting in the 1980's; when the patent expired after a number of years, some of the generic companies brought forth their own versions of Prozac (fluoxetine) which are supposed to be of the same chemical structure, but might be produced using a different technique or process; when there was only one (or two) generic versions of Prozac, the generic was less than branded Prozac, but still pricey; nowadays, generic Prozac is everywhere and costs less today. (2) When Paxil was poised to go generic, one of the generic companies started to sell generic Paxil (paroxetine) in the USA before the patent here had expired: there appeared to be two sets of opinions regarding the exact date of patent expiration. (3) Vivactil and Surmontil were never wildly popular and eventually went generic; at that time, not even the generic version(s) were selling well—Odyssey Pharmaceuticals bought the rights to produce the branded versions and was selling old drugs with expired patents as branded drugs and at branded prices! (in the USA, at least) (4) Eli Lilly makes Zyprexa, a very popular medication for Bipolar and Schizophrenia; while Zyprexa was still under patent protection in the USA, one of my uninsured patients was ordering generic Zyprexa (olanzapine) from India; I have no knowledge of international laws, but this would appear to be a case of some sort of piracy; so how does the patent-holder deal with this violation of international law? The unfortunate fact is that the seventeen years exclusivity sometimes starts ticking before the original medication debuts on the market, so that the original drug company sometimes has fewer than seventeen years in which to recoup its loss for R&D: this is the story of Wellbutrin in America. There are many such odd stories about generic and branded drugs.

BTC—behind the counter medication

CHRONIC—is a psychiatric disorder that lasts for years or decades (in general medicine, a chronic disease lasts over three months). In practice, chronic psychiatric patients are assumed to have a permanent condition

Controlled substance—see scheduled drug, DEA;

DEA—Drug Enforcement Administration (US government) has oversight over and controls every step in the manufacture, distribution, prescribing, and dispensing of addictive drugs and medications, such as amphetamines and Ritalin. The DEA can also control access to chemicals needed as precursors (ingredients) to make these drugs. The DEA possesses extensive police-like abilities to enforce the laws governing access to all dangerous drugs and addictive medications. The average doctor does not routinely have direct personal contact with the DEA, but if we do, then it is usually a solemn experience.

DEPRESSION-EQUIVALENT DISORDER—these are psychiatric conditions that are not Depression, but occur with high frequency in Depressive families: notably ADHD and compulsive disorders

(alcoholism, drug addiction, overeaters, gamblers, compulsive hoarders-shoppers-collectors)

DISCONTINUATION SYNDROME—see SSRI in List of Antidepressants (Part Three)

DOPAMINE—is considered to be one of the three main feel-good "brain hormones" with powerful antidepressant effects; it is related chemically to norepinephrine and adrenaline;

DSM—Diagnostic and Statistical Manual: is the official handbook used in America to diagnose psychiatric disorders; it is published and periodically updated by the APA; the current one is DSM-IV-TR (4th edition, text-revision); it provides no guidelines for therapies, however, and makes no treatment recommendations;

DYSPHORIA—see Introduction to Cycling Depression in Part Two

ECT—Electro-Convulsive Treatment, treatment for severe Depression typically using electricity ("shock treatment"); certain chemicals or insulin have also been used to induce the shock in the past;

EUPHORIA—see Introduction to Cycling Depression in Part Two

EUTHYMIA—see Introduction to Cycling Depression in Part Two

FDA—is the federal agency (Food and Drug Administration) that oversees the safety of foods and drugs (and other treatments and treatment devices) within the USA.

GENERIC DRUGS—see BRANDED DRUGS

HYPOMANIA—see Introduction to Cycling Depression in Part Two

LIMERENCE—the intense state of early passionate obsession in a serious romance

MANIA—see Introduction to Cycling Depression in Part Two

MEDICATION—refers to prescription medicines (R_x medicines)

MELANCHOLY (Melancholia)—see Introduction to Cycling Depression in Part Two

Noradrenaline—see norepinephrine

NOREPINEPHRINE—is presumed to be one of the three main "feel-good" "brain hormones"; it is closely related to adrenaline and dopamine; see Brain Hormone above; in this book, I am preferentially using "norepinephrine" (instead of "noradrenaline") and "adrenaline" (instead of "epinephrine");

OTC—these are medications sold Over The Counter (without a prescription)

"PURIFIED MEDICATION" refers to two different concepts, the proper chemical terms for which are (1) "active metabolites" and (2) "enantiomers": (1) an "active metabolite" is a "daughter medication" that may have fewer side effects and may provide much of the antidepressant effect—the active metabolite is a "stripped-down" by-product of the original oral pill, and is typically produced in the liver after the pill is swallowed; for example Pamelor is the active metabolite of Elavil: Joan swallows Elavil which goes to the liver (where a carbon/methyl group is stripped off) it is turned into Pamelor which accounts for more of the antidepressant effect than the original pill of Elavil; (2) as far as enantiomers, most medications will crystallize into two mirror images like identical twins, except that one is the "bad twin" (annoying side effects) and the other is the "good twin" (desirable antidepressant effects), for example Lexapro is the enantiomer of Celexa, and Pristiq, is from Effexor;

PROVIDER—refers to any mental health professional who provides service: psychiatrists, psychologists, counselors, psychoanalysts, and psychotherapists ("therapists")

PSYCHOSTIMULANT—see stimulants

PTSD—is a very serious type of Anxiety Disorder that can be caused by catastrophic stress;

Rx—any medication sold on prescription (that is not OTC, BTC, or Schedule VI)

RESTLESS LEG SYNDROME—(RLS) is being recognized nowadays as a common source of sleep disturbance. It is twice as common in women and may be aggravated by certain medications, including certain antidepressants (given at bedtime). The symptoms include a need to move the legs at night, thus interrupting sleep slightly; immobility can cause the legs to feel restless; moving the legs can relieve the symptoms for a while. There are several other common causes of nighttime leg movements and muscle cramps; these symptoms should be discussed with a doctor familiar in treating these types of disorders, preferably a neurologist. There are two FDA-approved medications for RLS and both of them are Parkinson's medications, which are usually prescribed by neurologists or neuropsychiatrists. I may try giving my patients Seroquel or Neurontin (which usually help RLS), and if this is not successful, I will suggest they see a neurologist. Seroquel and Neurontin are not FDA-approved for RLS, but can still be tried as an "off-label" treatment (this is not unethical or illegal).

RUPD—Recurrent Unipolar Depression: see Cycling Depression in Part Two

Scheduled drugs—are considered to be dangerous or addicting drugs, or both dangerous and addicting; this status is apparent because these drugs are not just Rx, but also scheduled; any scheduled drug is in one (or two) of these six categories: C-I, C-II, C-III, C-IV, C-V, or C-VI, where C-I would be pronounced as "Schedule One"; (some drugs are in two separate categories depending upon their use and compounding: GHB and cocaine, for example); the DEA is in charge of monitoring every aspect of the production, distribution, and consumption of these drugs; access to the drug is controlled by the DEA and restricted by doctors' prescriptions

SEROTONIN—one of the three main "feel-good" "brain hormones" with antidepressant effect, presumably; Prozac was the first medication with potent serotonin effect that was recognized as such, and Prozac thus became the first SSRI antidepressant; see "brain hormone"

Somatizing—some patients have a "non-emotional" Depression, that feels like a physical illness of the body; these patients are unaware of their Depression and think that they have a real medical problem in their bodies: this is called "somatizing" ("soma" means "body" in Greek): examples of somatizing symptoms are: vague miserable and lousy feelings, mild backache (too much time lying in bed or sitting in tension at the workplace), stomach acidity (worrying), headaches (stress), flare-up of asthma (emotions), and so on. These patients think their symptoms are in their bodies and not in their heads. Family doctors think that the symptoms are in the patients' heads and not in their bodies. The truth is that all symptoms are processed in the brain, so in a sense, all symptoms of all diseases are always [sensed and interpreted] in the head. Family doctors see a lot of mildly Depressed people who are somatizing—these patients are Depressed, but they do not realize it. Sometimes the family doctors do not realize it, either, for the first few visits. Family doctors end up treating a lot of mild Depressives.

Stimulant Antidepressants—also called Psychostimulants; this is a hot topic nowadays; these drugs were designed as a modified form of adrenaline in the hopes of producing an adrenaline-like drug to make people lively; the result was *amphetamines, the first antidepressants* ever discovered (a century ago). And, their first medicinal use was specifically to eliminate Depression and fatigue by producing euphoria and motivation—and they do this very well. However, the antidepressant effect lasts only during the day; they are imperfect antidepressants when compared to non-addicting antidepressants that provide long-term relief for weeks or months or years, not just for a few hours every day; people who take amphetamines in the morning feel lively for several hours, but usually "come down" or "crash" by evening. Stimulants were popular during World War II (Hitler and the Nazis took huge doses as did we and Japan). The drugs became popular here after World War II when Americans expanded the use of the drugs beyond mere treatment of Depression, and began also to use them for performance-enhancement (working faster, competing harder) and cognitive-enhancement (thinking smarter). With habitual use of these drugs, people, in general, become driven, hardworking, and successful, but some people also set themselves up for addiction, premature heart disease, strokes, and suicidal Depression. In the third wave, Americans used these pills as "diet pills," and we thought that they were excellent weight-loss medications. Unfortunately, over the next decades, it became apparent that pills will not cure obesity. Americans are once again clamoring for expanded access to these drugs, and we are now in the fourth wave of finding new uses for stimulants. This time around, and under the studied guidance of the Pharmaceutical Industry, the drugs are touted as a treatment for Adult ADHD. Curiously, most adults now taking them never had ADHD, which is a childhood disease that begins before age seven, thus casting a cloud of suspicion upon the contemporary explosion in Adult ADHD diagnoses. Many of these adults have a form of Depression or "job fatigue," so perhaps we should give them a realistic diagnosis of Depression and Occupational Problem (this is a real diagnosis, code V62.2) instead of contriving a pseudo-diagnosis of Adult ADHD. Another group of adults are impulsive and compulsive and want to use these drugs to feel good and to live life in the fast lane; these are the "Jimmy Dean" people: 'live hard, die young, leave a beautiful corpse'. They want stimulants and they want them NOW! They apparently object to a "nanny government" that is telling them how to live (and die). On the one hand, if we make these drugs available to all adults who want them, then we will raise our national productivity (GDP). Ironically, on the other hand, the "Jimmy Dean's" may pay dearly: they may pay much money (FICA) into their social security retirement fund (SSI), that they will never live to collect. However, a lot of them will survive their amphetamine-induced strokes and heart attacks and end up permanently disabled (SSD) as young adults. People like Rhonda, who become addicted to the drugs, will have serious problems. On the other hand, it is true that some people in every society will always become addicted to some chemical—whichever chemical is available then and there. Stimulants are all addicting drugs subject to strict control by the DEA: amphetamines, Ritalin, Cylert, and several others. These drugs are also made and sold illegally on the street where they command a high price. In rare cases, stimulants may be used to treat certain forms of Depression (see Phyllis' story in Part Two).

APPENDIX ONE

This appendix explains how I generated fifteen types of Depression from the original seven types. In order to understand Appendix One, please read the last Sections of Part One and when at the very end of Section One, continue reading below. After finishing Appendix One, go directly to the beginning of Part Two.

...So, if we make a list incorporating these above variables, we will have:

CAUSES and RISK FACTORS (explained earlier in Part One)
- Unknown causes
- Known causes
- Risk Factors

SEVERITY
- Mild
- Moderate
- Severe
- Severely Psychotic

DURATION
- Brief (months)
- Intermediate duration (a year or two)
- Long-lasting (a few to several years)
- Permanent (chronic)

TREATABILITY

- Easy to treat
- Hard to treat
- Treatment failure

OCCURRENCE

- Occurs only once
- Recurrent (Occurs more than once)
- appears unpredictably
- appears cyclically as moods in well-defined "up" and "down" cycles, like a sine wave
- appears predictably: after every baby is born; with every winter;
- Occurs once and then stays the same: it becomes chronic (permanent)

We can now apply these variables to our simple list of Depressions to generate and explain the seven basic types of Depression:

SEVEN TYPES of Depression

- Reactive Depression
- Minor Depression
- Dysthymia
- Major Depression
- Cycling Depressions
- Other Depressions
- Secondary Depressions

We can start off simply by applying the variables to describe the seven basic types of Depressions:

- Mild, easy to treat, brief, known cause = Reactive Depression
- Mild, easy, brief, unknown cause = Minor Depression
- Mild, easy, long-lasting = Dysthymia
- Moderate, easy, intermediate duration = moderate Major Depression
- Moderate, hard to treat, cyclic = Cyclic Depressions
- Mild, easy, predictable/periodic, known cause = Other Depression (Winter Depression)

271

- Moderate, known cause = Secondary Depression (Alcoholic Depression)

However, as I had stated previously, there are actually many types of Depression. We can increase our list of variables to include a description of how Depressed the mood is. The mood in Depression can be mildly, moderately, or severely Depressed:

DEGREE of MOOD Depression
- Mildly Depressed mood
- Moderately Depressed mood
- Severely Depressed mood
- Severely Depressed psychotic mood

And we can specify if the mood is constantly Depressed with the same degree of Depressed mood that remains the same year in and year out: this is the mood in a chronic Depression:
- Chronically Depressed mood: people with a chronically Depressed mood can have
- mildly chronically Depressed mood
- moderately chronically Depressed mood, or
- severely chronically Depressed mood

So now, if we apply our DEGREES of Mood Depression to the SEVEN TYPES of Depression, we can generate an expanded list of the seven types of Depression:

- Mild, easy to treat, brief, known cause = Reactive Depression
- Mild, easy, brief, unknown cause = Minor Depression
- Mild, easy to treat, long-lasting = Dysthymia
- Mild, easy, intermediate duration = mild Major Depression
- Mild-moderate, hard to treat, long-lasting = Chronic Depression
- Moderate, easy, intermediate duration = moderate Major Depression
- Moderate, hard, long-lasting, recurrent = recurrent Major Depression

- Severe, difficult to treat, long-lasting = severe Major Depression
- Very severe, hard to treat, long-lasting = Severe Psychotic Major Depression
- Moderate, hard to treat, cyclic = Bipolar Depression
- Severe, hard to treat, cyclic = Manic Depression
- Moderate, hard, brief-intermediate, periodic = Bipolar Depression (Borderline)
- Mild, easy, periodic, known cause = Other Depression (Winter Depression)
- Moderate, known cause = Secondary Depression (Alcoholic Depression)
- Very Severe, brief, treatment failure = suicide

In this way, we can go further to generate an expanded list of fifteen types of Depression from the **basic seven** (shown below in **bold type**). This will suit the purposes of the book as we study patients in Part Two. Here is the expanded list of fifteen main types of Depression (*examples and explanations of the corresponding Depressions are shown inside parentheses*):

- **Reactive Depression**
- **Minor Depression**
- **Dysthymia**
- **Major Depression**:
- *Mild Major Depression*
- *Moderate Major Depression*
- *Chronic Depression*
- *Severe (Major) Depression*
- *Severe (Major) Psychotic Depression*
- **Cycling Depressions**:
- *Bipolar Depression*
- *Borderline Depression (with Dysphoria)*
- *Manic Depression*
- *Cyclothymia*
- *Recurrent Unipolar Depression (a type of major Depression that cycles)*
- **Other Depressions**: Winter Depression, post-partum Depression, and Grief Depression (*Prolonged Grief*)

- **Secondary Depressions** are due to Medical Illness, Drug Addiction, Alcoholism, or Addiction to Prescription Pills: *Depression due to Multiple Sclerosis, Alcoholic Depression, Depression due to Amphetamines, Depression due to Prescription Drugs, Depression associated with Child Abuse*

Further Explanation of the examples and explanations inside parentheses: The names of psychiatric conditions have changed over the last two centuries. We periodically rename the disorders. However, the disorders remain the same and the treatment remains the same. The reasons for these name changes are numerous. I have tried to avoid using more than one name for a condition while trying to expose the reader to the contemporary names. The one problem with this approach is that most of the older names are easier to recognize and understand, and these names are more descriptive, whereas the new names are often wordy and lengthy. For example, Reactive Depression is one type of a minor Depression that occurs as a bad reaction to an unpleasant stress. This name is very descriptive and easy to remember and understand: it is a bad reaction to a stress factor that results in making people Depressed, hence Reactive Depression. However, the American Psychiatric Association (APA) has formally renamed Reactive Depression as "Adjustment Disorder with Depressed Mood"; and if that weren't bad enough, if it occurs with anxiety symptoms also, then it is called "Adjustment Disorder with Mixed Anxiety and Depressed Mood." This diagnosis contains eight words and is longer than a simple sentence. Clearly, I have no intention of burdening the reader with such a highfalutin' term. Some other countries may still be using the term "Reactive Depression," and American psychiatrists may use this term in casual conversation. Situational Depression was another minor Depression that was caused by an unpleasant situation. Situational Depression is therefore like a Reactive Depression, and we used these terms almost interchangeably in the past, but neither one is a formal official diagnosis in America anymore (the formal official diagnosis must be used in order for the doctor to be paid).

Likewise, the APA has renamed Minor Depression as "Depressive Disorder Not Otherwise Stated." We need five words to describe it!

Psychotic Depression is obviously a severe Depression in which the patient is also psychotic; the APA has likewise renamed this condition as

"Severe Major Depression with Mood-Congruent Psychotic Features."
All other such examples appear in the list as printed (*inside parentheses*
and in *italics*). These are all good examples of technical jargon. The stated
reason for changing these names is to make them more statistically
valid, but they also become less "user-friendly" and much harder to
teach to the casual reader.

The reader does not need to memorize this list of fifteen types of
Depression. I just want to provide a basic framework for understanding
how badly some people feel and why. So, armed with this information,
let's plunge ahead into Part Two that deals with realistic stories of
fictitious patients.